THE CARBOHYDRATE EFFECT

JUST PERHAPS?

aims to celebrate the work of pioneering doctors
who have dedicated their lives to an aspect of medical
practice that lies outside the mainstream yet
which – just perhaps – has something of
vital importance to offer us.

The Carbohydrate Effect

A tribute to Dr Wolfgang Lutz

Valerie Bracken

JUST PERHAPS?

EDINBURGH

3

Books by Valerie Bracken:
My Life without Bread: Dr Lutz at 90 (2014)
Dr Lutz and his Chickens: Carbohydrate and Arterial Health (2019)
The Art of Everyday Movement: A Handbook for Women
Dr Bess Mensendieck (translated and edited by Valerie Bracken) (2020)
Our Friend the Cabbage Leaf: The Work of Dr Anselme Blanc (2022)

The Carbohydrate Effect: A Tribute to Dr Wolfgang Lutz
Copyright © Valerie Bracken, 2023
All rights reserved
The moral right of the author has been asserted
First published in Great Britain in 2013 as Uncle Wolfi's Secret
Revised in 2016, third edition and retitled in 2023
www.justperhaps.co.uk
ISBN 9798388346001

Cover design by JUST PERHAPS?
Back cover painting by Charlotte Cornforth

INTRODUCTION

'Should carbohydrates form the mainstay of our diet? Are they the rightful main source of our energy? Does this actually fit with our heritage or with the inherent design of our bodies?', asks Dr Lutz, as he ponders the seeming erosion of our health by what he calls The Carbohydrate Effect.

Austrian-born: Dr Wolfgang Lutz (1913-2010) was an outstanding scientist and doctor of medicine, who became a consultant in Internal Medicine in his forties. Over the next fifty years, he carefully watched the outcome of carbohydrate restriction on himself and on his many patients.

I was privileged to have the help of Dr Lutz in understanding his ideas over a great many years. His thinking was challenging yet his method of treatment was straight-forward and effective. How could I share this with others in simple non-technical language? Perhaps through the simplicity of a child?

So I created a semi-fictional setting in which Dr Lutz became my 'Uncle Wolfi' and I, his inquisitive young 'niece', Sparrow who keeps asking very basic and probing questions.

The narrative and setting are imaginary, yet the exploration of ideas is genuine, as are the descriptions of the way the body works, of Dr Lutz himself, references to his therapeutic work and his suggested way of eating, to his books, his humour and his devotion to the wellbeing of his patients.

The Carbohydrate Effect (formerly Uncle Wolfi's Secret) describes the type of food to eat, supplies us with the tools to look critically at the many myths that abound in this field and explains why the observations made by Wolfgang Lutz are of fundamental importance to our health.

Valerie Bracken 2023

CONTENTS

Part I   My Uncle Wolfi

Part II   Wondering

Part III   'Doing a Wolfi'

PART I

MY UNCLE WOLFI

1 BY THE POND

I have always been fond of my Uncle Wolfi. Ever busy at some idea of his, he was still always ready to stop for a chat.

We used to laugh when he came to visit us in England, for every time we offered him a plate of chips with his fish, he would say:

"Thank you very much, I'll have two."

But Uncle Wolfi meant two chips, not two platefuls.

Uncle Wolfi has been a doctor for many, many years. When he was nearly 80 years old, he retired but soon started to work again. I remember Mum saying that he was not the sort to retire while there was still so much important work to be done.

The best times were in the holidays. Luckily for me, in the spring and summer Uncle always spent time in his home in the mountains of Austria.

Uncle Wolfi had a big house next to a lake and it is there that I spent so many memorable school holidays playing in his rambling old garden, a garden which had a large pond and an orchard, as well as every bush and plant imaginable.

He has always done a lot of thinking, has Uncle Wolfi. During these holidays, I often used to find him sitting by the huge pond in his garden. Sometimes I would see him staring into the water and at other times he would sit there quietly, shaking his head slowly and frowning.

Uncle did get grumpy at times, but on the whole he was a kindly old man and I liked him a lot.

One day, I asked him why he shook his head and frowned.
Uncle looked up and smiled at my question. He paused for a
while and then he said softly:

"Oh, Sparrow, they just don't see!" Uncle Wolfi often called
me 'Sparrow' and it had become my nickname.

"Who don't?" I wondered.

"Oh they – the scientists, the medics, the journalists – more
or less all of them," he muttered. "They just don't see," he
repeated, looking again into the water.

"Don't see what, Uncle Wolfi?" I pursued, interrupting
his reverie in my eagerness.

Uncle Wolfi was again shaking his head and frowning.
Then he said something quite extraordinary:

"They don't see the importance of beginnings. They don't
see who or what we are, because they forget who and what we
were – and how on earth can they possibly know what we
need, if they don't see who we are!"

I didn't have a clue what he was talking about. Here, Uncle
caught hold of his frowns and tossed them away.

Then, turning to me, Uncle Wolfi continued more amicably:

"Well, let's put it this way – and I don't think I am wrong
in this – if we overlook the little that we do know about our
beginnings, there is no adequate anchorage for our reasoning
which, of course, soon goes adrift. Yes, maybe that's it."

I was still mystified.

Uncle remained thoughtful for what seemed like a long time.
His eyes had a faraway look as he resumed speaking:

"It may seem very strange to you, little one, but sometimes
when I look into my pond, it is as if I am seeing right back to
the beginning of time."

He said this so quietly and with such an air of mystery that I have been asking questions and listening to his stories ever since.

For I soon realised that Uncle Wolfi really did take notice of a bit of history that other people had forgotten, that he knew both important secrets and the origin of some of the secrets. I longed to know more.

Next time I saw Uncle by the pond, I ventured to ask what he saw as he gazed into the water. He didn't answer for many minutes. He just went on gazing.

At length, he said in a voice that seemed somehow changed:

"I see a time when there was no land on this planet of ours we call earth – a time when all was ocean, when there was little oxygen in the atmosphere of the earth and almost the only living things in existence were tiny organisms with only one cell . . ."

"But how could they breathe with so little oxygen?" I asked puzzled. We had done oxygen at school.

Uncle blinked a few times before answering:

"Oh, they didn't, not in the way you mean. They fermented rather than breathed."

"Like turning into alcohol?" I suggested.

Uncle sighed:

"No, more like the sort of fermenting that happens when we salt cabbage in a cask and then weigh it with a large stone to make sauerkraut."

"Yuk! Oh, how it must have smelled!"

Uncle made no comment, but sat silent for a while, turning his eyes once more to the pond.

"But to continue. I was talking about the days when there was just ocean and these tiny organisms with one cell were living and multiplying by dividing and fermenting in this 'primordial soup' as they call it."

And here he began to chuckle as if at a private joke.

"But what sort of soup was it, Uncle Wolfi?" I asked intrigued. My favourite was tomato, or maybe burnt onion, or just perhaps Mum's homemade oxtail.

"But that's just it!" exclaimed Uncle, still chuckling but not making any sense that I could see.

Without further explanation, he asked:

"Do you know how long ago that was? More than two billion years!" said Uncle Wolfi, answering his own question. "That means that though I personally have been on this earth a mere 80 years or so, there is a sense in which I stretch back over two billion years!"

His eyes twinkled as he looked at my uncomprehending and somewhat doubting face.

"Oh, there is a sense in which you stretch back that far, too," he said, laughing. "Your father and mother had a father and mother, who had a father and mother, who had a father and mother and so on back and back in time.

And then back in time further still, right back through different ancestral species and then back again as far as the one-celled creatures, then even before that to the very beginning of life on earth."

"When we were all swimming in seafood soup?" I asked hopefully, recalling the bouillabaisse I had eaten on a former holiday.

"Oh little one, be serious for a moment!"

But, remembering I knew nothing of those ancient days, Uncle added:

"The time I am talking about was a long, long time before there was anything so complicated as a fish."

Uncle Wolfi paused awhile, tossing a pebble into the pond.

"You know, even in our present lifetime, we start out in life as only one cell – one egg cell from our mother which starts dividing as soon as it is fertilised by our father's contribution.

Fortunately, we progress a little more rapidly! It may have taken something like two billion years for the human species to evolve from one-cell organisms, but now we are human, for us to go from one cell to a fully-formed baby with trillions of cells and ready to be born, it only takes around nine months.

Don't you think that's amazing? I'll tell you all about it one day," he promised. "Well, about some of it anyway."

"Trillions of cells," I repeated, awestruck.

"For now," he added, "just remember that there is always a sense in which we come out of what has gone before and, just as important, that there is always change along the way."

Then we went off together to gather raspberries and I felt a lot easier. Old people say some strange things.

2 APES

In Uncle Wolfi's garden, I used to play wonderful games.

There were mountains all around, which I could see if I stood up. But if I crouched down in the grass, the trees and bushes surrounded me like a tropical forest. I would imagine wild animals coming to take a drink in the large lake that was nearby.

Instantly I was an ape in the Africa of old, loping along the ground with other apes and emitting little grunting noises. Then I would climb contentedly into one of the gnarled old fruit trees in the search for food.

I remember playing this game towards the end of one summer holiday. I think I was about eight years old at the time. I was sitting in a tree as Uncle Wolfi came by on his regular half-hour walk and I scrambled down to join him.

"Up to monkey business again, I see," he said winking.

"I am playing ancestral relatives, actually," I replied a little stiffly. "I am not a little monkey as mother would have it. I am a great ape!" I announced proudly.

"Our ape-like ancestors lived millions of years ago," Uncle informed me. "And there have been a lot of changes since! They say that the modern chimpanzee developed from a shared ancestry with us way back when," continued Uncle Wolfi.

"Well, they still feel like our relatives," I said, remembering my visits to London Zoo.

"Then may I perhaps have the pleasure of addressing you as my little chimp?" he added with a slight bow of his head, but his eyes were laughing.

"All right, Uncle," I agreed cheerfully. "Then I can be a chimp up your tree!" I said, scrambling up again onto a branch to go on with my game.

"Uncle Wolfi," I called out as he was walking away, "I could have my tea up here. Please can I? I know chimps eat fruit, and Aunt Helen has some oranges in the fruit bowl."

Uncle stopped, turned round and came back.

"Of course you can. It is certainly better than having your roving chimp friends stripping the leaves and fruit from every tree in sight!

I will, I think, also provide some insects and a small mammal to make your tea more authentic," chuckled the big man at the foot of the tree.

"Oh, don't be revolting, Uncle Wolfi. Anyway, I thought chimps just ate fruit."

"Not all the time, they also eat leaves, shoots and roots, so I'll bring you some salad too – I'm afraid that is as close as we can get to the plant food of an equatorial forest – and a little meat for good measure."

"And bread and butter?" I queried.

"Let me see," teased Uncle Wolfi, "now bread comes from wheat, which is a grass seed, and grass seed is hardly the type of food that chimpanzees eat!

Anyway, as far as I know, chimps haven't learnt to cook.

As for butter, no, sorry, and you'll have to pass on the ice cream, too!"

So that is how I got my chimp tea up a tree: an orange, some salad and a bit of ham, and it didn't seem so very different from what the grown-ups were eating indoors around the table.

But then I still had a lot to learn.

14

Next morning at breakfast, I found a little heap of bean sprouts by my plate.

"But . . ." I protested, eyeing the cornflakes hopefully – I knew they had been bought in especially for me.

Uncle Wolfi shook his head.

"A glass of milk?" I suggested meekly.

Again Uncle shook his head. The smell of the bacon and eggs that the others were eating made my mouth water and Uncle Wolfi read my longing.

"Come on, play the game, my little chimp," he said encouragingly. "If bean sprouts are not to your liking, you can run along and find some gooseberries in the garden."

"Cream and sugar to go with them?" I asked, making one last try. Uncle looked at me with his head on one side.

"Personally, I have no knowledge of chimpanzees milking cows, nor of buying groceries for that matter. Run along now! If you are lucky, you might also find a ripe apple – they are almost ready – or some late raspberries."

Apart from a few gooseberries, I was not lucky. All I found were some rather hard, greenish and unappetising blackberries.

By lunchtime, I was getting decidedly hungry.

I sat in a huff, pulling gooseberry prickles out of my fingers, and looking disconsolately at my plate of crudités, whilst the family enjoyed braune Kraftsuppe, a brown meat soup that smelled of oxtail and reminded me of home.

I toyed with a carrot stick, while Aunt Helen and Uncle Wolfi tucked into roast chicken and mushrooms.

Sensing that my tears were not far away, Uncle pushed his plate towards me. Gratefully, I took a chicken leg.

After that, I helped myself to two rather large helpings of a wonderful pudding called Schokoladensoufflé, made from eggs and dark chocolate with morello cherries on top, not very sweet but infinitely delicious.

At this, Uncle frowned slightly.

"Meet me by the pond," was all he said.

Later that afternoon, I went down to the pond and Uncle was all smiles, but I wasn't smiling.

"You said there is always a sense in which we come out of what went before," I grumbled. "Well, I didn't find it much fun being a chimp.

I'd have given a lot for a piece of toast and a hot drink. I was starving! And how was I supposed to enjoy bean sprouts when you were all eating a proper breakfast?" I asked fretfully.

Uncle merely raised one eyebrow.

"I enjoyed the chicken," I conceded earnestly, "and the pudding was heavenly! Thank you, Uncle Wolfi."

Uncle nodded. He has a soft spot for Aunt Helen's puddings.

"So, what did you learn, I wonder?" he enquired.

I thought about this for a moment.

"I think chimps would go hungry living up here in Austria!"

"Not quite the tropical forest of your imagination then?" asked Uncle.

He didn't have to rub it in, did he!

"And have you thought what a chimp would eat in winter?"

It made me shudder just thinking about the cold and snow of all those mountains.

In fact, I was just on the point of deciding I would have to invent fire, when Uncle Wolfi asked:

"Do you still want to be a chimp then, my little ancestral relative?"

"I think," I answered slowly, "I would have to become a hunter to survive the winter, or maybe a shepherd and drive my sheep down to the valleys when it got colder."

I was also picturing a house with a warm fire in the daytime and a warm bed to sleep in at night, rather than a cold and frosty platform of twigs on the branches of a tree.

"So, living in this climate, will you settle for being human after all, do you think?" he asked, watching my face intently.

"I think so, Uncle Wolfi. I really do think so."

"Well, it sounds to me like you've moved on a few million years in one swift bit of realism about your surroundings!

You see, we were never really apes, as such! We may have had ancestors in common millions of years ago, but we humans had our own subsequent history. Separate paths, if you like.

Gradually adapting to changes in circumstances, the pre-gorilla eventually became a gorilla, the pre-chimp a chimp, but they never became human."

"So we were never chimps?"

"No, during the intervening time – they say four to seven million years – the apes went one way and we went ours."

"Never chimps!" I repeated.

Then Uncle Wolfi said something I didn't really understand until many years later:

"My advice to you, niece of mine, is very simple: never forget you are a human being and not a chimp!"

3 THE SECRET

The following summer, I was back at Uncle Wolfi's.

One day, while we were cleaning up the pond together, I began thinking about all those patients Uncle Wolfi had got well again. Mum said there were many thousands of grateful people whom Uncle had helped.

"How do you do it, Uncle Wolfi?" I asked all of a sudden.

"How do I clean ponds?" asked Uncle, raising his head and looking at me, frowning a little.

"No, no, Uncle. How do you get so many people well that have so many horrid things wrong with them? Is it a secret or can you tell me?" I wondered aloud.

Uncle Wolfi now burst into laughter.

"A secret, bless my soul, what next!" he said, continuing to chuckle. "Oh little one, my secret is as old as the hills – well almost!" he added as an afterthought.

Then Uncle Wolfi looked at me for a long time, as if weighing something up.

"If you really want to know, I'm only too happy to share my 'secret'. It's a nice day, what do you say, Sparrow, to taking out the boat?"

That was a wonderful idea. Uncle Wolfi had a rowing boat and I liked nothing better than sitting dangling my fingers in the water while Uncle rowed across the lake with his strong hands on the oars. It looked so easy when he did it!

So we went to the lake and I clambered in. Uncle pushed the boat off and rowed us smoothly into the centre of the lake, then put up his oars.

From here, we had a good view of the mountains all around. A bird swooped low over the water, then suddenly dipped down, catching a fish in its beak, and flew off still holding tight the wriggling fish.

A dragonfly hovered and then darted after its prey.

"Those creatures certainly know what they want for their dinner," Uncle Wolfi mused.

"Of course they do," said I.

"Quite so, of course they do," echoed Uncle smiling. He sat awhile gazing up at the snowy peaks.

"Have you ever wondered why dragonflies and birds know what to eat and we humans get ourselves in such a muddle – such a muddle that you even have lessons at school as to what you ought to want to put in your mouth?

Does that not strike you as strange?"

I must admit I had not thought about it quite like that.

"But Uncle, what about your secret?" I asked impatiently.

"Hush, child. Slowly, slowly! Some secrets, especially such very old secrets have to be discovered by each person anew. So perhaps I should start by putting a question to you?

We are sitting here on the lake in a rowing boat. Now, if this boat were a motorboat, would it matter what fuel we put in the engine?"

"Of course it would, silly!"

Uncle raised his eyebrows a little at the appellation 'silly', but continued unabashed:

"And if we put in the wrong fuel?"

I pulled a face of vague apprehension.

"Quite!" said Uncle, nodding in approval. "Now, remember I told you that there are not billions but trillions of cells in our bodies? I bet you didn't know that most of these cells have their own little engines and sometimes many of them!"

Uncle was watching my expression of part amazement and part disbelief:

"Just think: these trillions of little engines all need fuel! It is all part of their design – like an outboard motor, only more complicated. Perhaps these little cell engines work best on the right amount and type of fuel?

What do you say to that idea, Sparrow?"

I sat silent: I was thinking of all those little engines.

Uncle Wolfi, too, said nothing but picked up the oars and rowed on for a time. After many minutes he spoke as if to himself:

"All those drugs and all that surgery, necessary sometimes, yet it seldom gets to the root of the problem!

But, you see, I had this grand idea – a brain-wave perhaps – that if I made certain changes to my patients' food supply, if I gave them a different and more suitable mix of foodstuffs, as it were, then this might give them a better internal mix of fuel, as well as giving them better raw materials for their bodies to work with.

By doing this, I hoped that all their body systems would then work more efficiently. Following from that, their bodies might start healing themselves and my patients would start to get better, only occasionally needing drugs or surgery.

And – Gott sei Dank – this is what usually happened!"

When Uncle started speaking about his medical work, his face changed: it lost that special smile of his, half teasing, half slightly mocking as though he could see a joke that others couldn't see.

He almost became a different person, all seriousness and concern. He was like that now and his look was searching, yet kindly. I was in awe of him at these times.

"Ah, little one," he said, bringing himself quickly back to the present moment.

Greatly puzzled, I was examining my hands.

"But Uncle Wolfi, I can't see or feel any engines!"

"No, you won't," said Uncle laughing. "They are minuscule, but they are there all the same, right inside you."

"But not real engines!"

"In essence, yes, they are little motors: they are miniature powerhouses, if you like."

"But what are they all for?" I asked intrigued.

"Simply to convert fuel to provide the energy we need for what goes on inside of us and, naturally, also for our daily lives in general.

Raising your arm to comb your hair or brush your teeth needs energy, you know," he added, "or staying warm or digesting a meal. Even thinking takes energy!"

I thought about that one.

"Take movement," he went on. "Everything that moves needs fuel converted to energy to enable motion: if I row, it is my energy that is used, if I sit still in a motorboat, we fetch in the fuel for it from outside.

Obviously, birds and dragonflies cannot go to a garage for their fuel so they have to make it from the food they eat. It works very well for them, it seems," concluded Uncle.

\ Right on cue, back came our dragonfly, darting past us, chasing something only it could see.

I began to understand something of Uncle's drift.

"Uncle Wolfi, I know you are right about food as fuel which we then convert into energy because, if I eat sweeties, I keep jumping up and down!"

"Hmm! Very probably," said Uncle with a sigh. "Yes, we eat to supply us with fuel and we also eat to supply us with what we need to repair and maintain our bodies and, of course, you young ones need building materials with which to grow big and strong."

"I eat because it's yummy and because my tummy rumbles if I don't."

Then, having been reminded of food and giving a little anticipatory bounce, I added:

"Oh, is it biscuit time?"

"Sit still or you'll rock the boat!" snapped Uncle. "Anyway, it's time we were heading for the shore."

Uncle's face had become grave, so I changed tack.

"Seriously, Uncle, you say that the dragonflies have their own food on which they keep well."

"That dragonflies eat mosquitoes and wasps, you mean? Yes, it would seem that given the right circumstances and the right surroundings, each type of living thing is endowed with the wherewithal – and this includes the know-how – to survive and thrive and multiply.

Part of this wherewithal is the right type of digestive system needed to deal effectively with its food, as well as the skill in catching it!"

His hand imitated the darting down of the dragonfly swiftly seizing its prey.

"The know-how is partly inborn, partly learnt. If, say, a butterfly's young can only thrive on a particular type of plant – and sometimes the right surroundings are very precise – then the butterfly will take care to lay her eggs on that particular type of plant.

In this way, the caterpillar not only has the food it needs but, when it eventually becomes a butterfly itself, it knows where to lay its own eggs: perhaps home is the leaf of a stinging nettle," he mused. "Now as for dragonflies . . ."

But I was getting impatient and broke in:

"I've got it, Uncle! You put your patients on their very own dragonfly diet and, and," I went on, trying to contain my excitement, "and, hey presto, they get well!"

"That is not how I would put it, child," he remarked dryly.

Uncle always called me child when he wanted to rebuke me:

"And I do not believe in magic. Hey presto, indeed! As if I snapped my fingers and people got well! Getting well can take a great deal longer than that."

"But what I mean, Uncle Wolfi, is that just because we are human doesn't mean that there isn't food that is right for us, food that will both keep our little engines ticking over contentedly and also provide the right raw materials for us to repair ourselves and so to get well.

Is that it? And that will help me grow big and strong," I added as an afterthought to show I really had been listening.

A smile came over Uncle's face, as he helped me out of the boat and tied it to its mooring.

"I think you are beginning to get an inkling of my secret. Well done!" he said, as we walked back to the house.

"But what? But which?" I burst out.

"And I think," continued Uncle Wolfi, unperturbed by my wild enthusiasm, "that you are starting out on a long and hopefully fascinating journey of discovery.

May I accompany you? It would give me great pleasure."

I nodded, speechless with joy.

"I can see we need a little history lesson to get a perspective on all this, and perhaps a little biology, too."

We reached the doorstep of the house. Uncle had a meeting to go to and I would be leaving for England before he returned.

"So, Aufwiedersehen, my little Fräulein!" he said, turning to me. "Until we meet again!"

To my surprise, Uncle Wolfi held out his right hand and we shook hands. It made me feel very grown-up.

4 OLD BONES

I did a lot of thinking that year. When at last the next summer holidays came round, I soon sought out Uncle in the lounge. Uncle Wolfi had been listening to opera on his record-player and was in mellow mood. He looked up at my eager face.

"Get your shoes on, Sparrow, and wait for me in the porch! It's time for my walk."

We were soon outside and we stood for a while, looking up at the high mountains.

"Many of the lower slopes are still forested, as you can see, but imagine all this area being covered with forest. It used to be that way once. How magnificent it must have been!

But it got too cold even for trees," he said, shaking his head. "And it was a long, long time ago."

I was bursting with questions, but Uncle insisted that we first walked down to the edge of the lake.

We found a nice open spot on the bank amidst lovely alpine flowers. From here, we could see the grassy slopes on the side of one of the mountains where lambs played together whilst their mothers ate steadily, seeming to take no notice of the games their young ones were playing. Nearby I could see the brilliant colours of a male pheasant, pecking for grubs; on the far side of the lake, cattle were lowing and clanking their bells.

At length, Uncle Wolfi spoke:

"I seem to remember you were suggesting that, perhaps, just as the bird and the dragonfly have their own foods, we too have our own way of eating, which suits the way our bodies work?"

"Oh yes, I did say that, but I can't think what it would be,"
I said picturing to myself one of the jam-packed shelves in our
local supermarket back home. "There is so much to choose
from. And I know my Mum says the ads on TV try to trick us
into believing nonsense.

It's easier for dragonflies!" I reflected, pouting slightly.

"Well, let's try and make it easier for ourselves. Let's play a
little game." That sounded more like it. I was full of curiosity
and ready for off.

"Shall we begin?" asked Uncle, making himself comfortable
on the grass. "Let us go back in time about 40,000 years – by
then we had long since developed into proper human beings.

We have just arrived in this part of the world and are living
as nomads at the edge of great ice sheets."

"Ice sheets like glaciers?" I asked.

"Like glaciers spreading as far as the eye could see! And we
are intelligent, tall, strong and healthy," continued Uncle.

"OK," I replied.

"What shall we have for lunch, niece of mine?"

Here Uncle spread out his arm to encompass the surrounding
landscape.

"Oh Uncle Wolfi, you are joking!"

"Of course, but indulge me in my little joke."

"I'll try!"

I looked around with fresh eyes. It was actually quite bleak
once you got away from Uncle's garden: just rough grass,
moss, rocks and a few scraggy bushes.

There were no fields of cabbages or cauliflowers, no
greenhouses or polytunnels, no orchards or even fields with
hedges round. It wasn't a bit like it was at home.

"It must have looked a bit like this in those days, don't you think, Sparrow? Colder perhaps, but the same sort of bare rocky mountainsides: possibly a few goats rather than sheep, but essentially the same.

There were a good few years to go before this whole area was completely covered in ice, sometimes incredibly deep."

"So, lunch?" asked Uncle, raising one eyebrow.

I was ready for him:

"What about roast lamb?" I said, glancing up at the sheep on the mountainside and adding as an afterthought, "preferably with chips and mint sauce. Do you think our early relatives ate potatoes, Uncle Wolfi?"

"Much too early for potatoes," replied he, "but we might be lucky with a little mint. I know there is some water mint further along the lake.

And it might have to be roast venison: it depends what we can find – and what we can catch!"

I hadn't thought about that aspect of lunch! Thinking of food, I reached into my pocket for some sweets, but Uncle stayed my hand.

"Oh, no, no food until we have caught that deer, and that might take a few days! I daresay the wild ancestors of those sheep would be tricky to catch, too. Very fleet of foot!"

Now that sounded terrible.

"But Uncle, if I had to wait so long for food, I would get quite faint," I objected.

"Not if you'd had a good hunk of game inside you recently."

I thought he wasn't serious, but he seemed to be.

"You see, we are organised so that our energy is constant, even if our food supply is intermittent," Uncle explained.

"My energy doesn't even last from breakfast to lunchtime," I said mournfully.

"Perhaps you are running on reserve? Too many afters and not enough main course?" he suggested mildly. "Think about it: if people felt faint after just missing a couple of meals, how could they go on hunting if they missed their prey? Or even sit patiently and alert by a seal hole for three days?"

I didn't fancy seal meat, but I tried to be brave:

"Perhaps, we could have some fish instead?" I suggested hopefully.

"Fish is thought to have come into our diet by then," said Uncle, considering the idea, "so yes, you shall have fish. Good idea. There's plenty in the lake.

Perhaps you would like to catch one while I light a fire?"

So, fish it would have to be, and maybe roast venison or the meat of an early type of sheep or goat for supper: that is if we were lucky.

I looked around for some vegetables to go with the fish. There was nothing obviously edible. I looked around for some fruit for dessert. Again there was nothing in sight.

"Not a lot of fruit and vegetables," I muttered.

"Not a lot of fruit and vegetables," echoed Uncle Wolfi.

"But you said we were intelligent, strong and healthy," I protested. "Could we really be intelligent, strong and healthy just on roast mutton and the odd mint leaf?"

"Indeed we could," said Uncle Wolfi, "and indeed we were, give or take a reindeer or two, or the odd woolly mammoth."

And before I could say another word, he raised his eyebrows and again said:

"Lunch?"

This time, forgetting all about history, we both happily tucked into the spare ribs with barbecue sauce which Uncle had so thoughtfully brought with him in a lunch box.

"Seriously though, Uncle," I said as soon as we had finished our food, "you don't actually mean that we could be healthy just on meat?"

"Naturally, where we live and in the modern age, it is not necessary to do so but think of living up here in the old days. Take our ancestors . . . "

"Have our ancestors always lived in these mountains?" I interrupted, imagining our family going back and back in time.

"Oh, it got far too cold for that at times. People living here then would have had to follow the animals south. Perhaps, as the weather got warmer again, they returned. I like to think so.

"It would seem strange with no people here!" I agreed.

"The climate here has changed a lot over the millennia, and so have the various types of plants and animals that have lived in these parts.

Did you know that, during the hot spells, elephants used to live here? And cave lions and grizzly bears?"

"What! Lions and elephants," I gasped in surprise.

"But that was way before the time we are talking about."

"But to answer your question about our ancestors," said Uncle after a pause. "Yes, groups of our most immediate predecessors – before we finally became human beings, that is – roamed around in this area for thousands of years, maybe 200,000 years according to some old bones that were found.

And it seems these predecessors of ours lived entirely on animal food, both the lean and the fat. You see, animal food gave them all they needed.

It was a clever arrangement: they let the grazing animals do the digesting of the moss, lichen and grass – the insides of these animals had special arrangements which enabled them to do this comfortably – and then they ate the grazers.

This suited the tummies of our ancestors very well!

And have our tummies changed much since those days? I doubt it," he concluded.

Uncle Wolfi was opening a whole new world to me. I had only seen lions in the zoo, but here I was sitting on the very spot where lions might have been devouring their dinner!

And then our own predecessors, a great many thousands of years ago, were here eating a very similar dinner!

It was difficult to believe: it was so like something out of a fairy tale!

Even our own kin of 40,000 years ago might have been right here at the edge of the lake, making a fire to roast their fish or their lamb with a sprig of water mint, just like Uncle Wolfi and I were contemplating doing.

Such fare was enough, Uncle said, to make them big and strong – strong enough to withstand the cold and the ice.

I stretched out on the grass and thoughtfully chewed a grass stalk. I eyed the pheasant, which eyed me as if saying:

"Your uncle is right, you know! Mother nature plans things very well! See what fine feathers I grow on a diet of grubs, shoots and insects!"

I am sure it winked.

5   LONG, LONG AGO

The following Easter, I was back at Uncle Wolfi's.

The mountains were white and glistening in the pale sunshine as Uncle and I took a walk along the lakeshore. Easter was late that year. The snow lower down the mountain slopes was already beginning to melt. I enjoyed the crackle underfoot of the icy particles that still lingered in the grass.

"Uncle," I exclaimed, jumping with delight in a slushy bit of snow, "what did you mean when you said that there is always a sense in which we come out of what has gone before?"

"Just that, biologically-speaking, what we were matters to what we are now," he replied as he walked on.

"But Uncle," I objected, running to catch up with him, "you said that I was never to forget I was a human and not a chimp."

"That is also true," he replied simply, "and that is because of the importance of all that happened in between."

"Oh Uncle, you do talk in riddles!"

I wished the snow were crisper so I could make a snowball. But I pretended to throw one at him. He ducked, laughing, and held out a placating hand, which I took.

"Uncle, you do make it hard for me to understand."

"Perhaps if I talk in riddles," he suggested soothingly, "I do this for you to have a chance of teasing out my meaning?"

I was getting nowhere.

"Let me try you with something very straightforward, Uncle Wolfi. Take food: what do you think we should eat?"

"It is a very modern concept this business of what we should eat. For the greater part of our history, the question has been, not what we should eat, but what we could actually find to eat. Choice seldom came into it."

"But that apart, Uncle, what do you, yourself, recommend? And don't joke about woolly mammoths this time, please," I pleaded, "or rhino steaks! I'm serious."

Uncle Wolfi did his best to look serious, too.

"Well, now, let me see. Not counting woolly mammoths or rhinos, I would say that the safest food is still any that has been part of our diet for at least 100,000 years."

"So what was available for our nomadic ancestors to eat? Even forty thousand years ago, in this area of Austria it would have to be food from the animal kingdom: animals, birds, insects and perhaps the occasional egg and, for some people, there would be fish."

"So, bacon and egg for breakfast would be fine," I said thankfully.

"Wild boar and, at certain times of year, an egg, why not!"

"And, Uncle Wolfi, can I have cheese on toast for lunch?" I asked earnestly.

"Well, milk, butter, yoghurt and cheese, in other words the food of the herders and domesticators, only entered our food supply during the last 10,000 years or so.

"They are comparatively recent foods, but I suppose you may, Sparrow, if cheese on toast takes your fancy."

"However, we must bear in mind that this later period begins to present a few challenges: first cereal, which was also a new arrival, later on sugar and then the ready-prepared commercial foods of the last fifty to a hundred years!"

"Oh, Uncle, I asked you what I should eat!" I remonstrated.

"My apologies, have I not answered you? I was just putting things into a sort of general perspective, a rule of thumb to go by. Start with the bigger picture, the grand canvas," he added, smiling to himself.

At this point I skidded on an icy patch under the slush and Uncle suggested we climb a bit higher to where the snow was still crisp and our footing would be more secure. We made our way cautiously further up.

"I can see that it makes sense for our food to come from our immediate surroundings – in those days, as you say, there was no option – and that it makes sense to move around looking for food – ditto," I slowly conceded. "I can see that if you lived where there was a lot of snow and ice, there probably wouldn't be much plant food."

Here we paused. The high mountains all around us were spectacular, so much whiteness yet with big splashes of greys and blues and purples. I could see the whole expanse of the lake and its shores.

I saw nothing move, no obvious wildlife other than a solitary raptor circling far overhead and then hovering. What had it seen with its marvellous eyesight that I could not see: a mountain hare, perhaps? But no, it didn't swoop but flew on. Uncle, too, had been gazing up at it.

"Wonderful birds, aren't they!" he exclaimed.

There was a well-demarcated path, so we walked on a little.

"Yet Uncle Wolfi," I said, returning to the question I had been wondering about, "if we can buy any food we want at the supermarket, why does all this matter?"

I felt it was a good point.

"And from any part of the world," I added, feeling a little proud of my observation.

"As I said," replied Uncle calmly, "it matters because of who or what we are."

"More riddles! But Uncle, the lot before us – our 'immediate predecessors' I think you called them – may have roamed over half the globe, but they did die out, didn't they.

In fact, the lot before them died out, too.

Do you think it was because they ate so much meat?" I asked with seeming innocence, adding:

"I mean, they must have been terribly ill, all that meat and no fruit and veg!"

Uncle Wolfi laughed out loud and his eyes twinkled with merriment. He had a special way of laughing, did Uncle Wolfi.

"On the contrary," he said at length, "to survive extreme climatic conditions, they had to be very fit and well. No, the 'lot before us', as you so disrespectfully put it, were a sturdy lot and enough of them did survive and breed to be around on this earth for a longer period of time than we humans have been here so far."

"But . . . " was all I could utter at the time.

"As to dying out, they probably vanished for several valid reasons.

Firstly, living by hunting is a risky business, for what if the bison or reindeer herd doesn't come by one year and a whole group simply can't find food?"

I thought of the bird of prey that didn't get its dinner just now.

"Secondly, for many years – maybe 5,000 or so – both we and they were living in this area at the same time: perhaps we were not too friendly towards them? We don't know."

34

"I know that cavemen had clubs!" I said, remembering comic strips of our savage ancestors wielding big spiky clubs and dragging their womenfolk by the hair.

"It seems, though, that there was some intermarriage," continued Uncle Wolfi regardless, "in which case they didn't exactly vanish.

Just look at any large crowd of people nowadays and you will see one or two people carrying reminders of them with their jutting eyebrows, the flattened top of the head, the short neck and head poked forwards. In fact, it is highly probable that I have some of their genes in me – and you, too, Sparrow!"

"Me?" I queried, a little worried.

I looked up at Uncle who was tall, slim and upright. He wasn't that shape, but maybe I was? I put my hand on the crown of my head to check.

"But, you know, it is nothing to worry about, little one, rather something to be proud of. After all, they had very big brains!" said Uncle, smiling.

I remained silent for a while and then spoke:

"You say they ate nothing but meat and fat?"

"True. It seems so anyway," said Uncle.

"Are you suggesting that it was all that meat and fat that made their brains grow so big?"

"I'm not suggesting anything. People must work that one out for themselves. Though perhaps," said Uncle thoughtfully, "perhaps it was precisely the meat-eating of our predecessors that helped give rise to us, that is: helped make us into the modern humans we are?

What do you think, Sparrow?"

Was Uncle Wolfi teasing, I wondered?

35

"What is certain is that without our ancestors, there would be no us!" concluded Uncle Wolfi.

"What we were, matters to what we are now," I quoted, for I had learnt Uncle's little sayings by heart.

"Exactly so," nodded Uncle. "But let us look at this another way. Now, what if that one type of leaf our caterpillar could feed on was suddenly not available? We've agreed the butterfly would go further afield searching for it. But what if that type of leaf no longer existed?"

"It would be scuppered," I said, "like the pandas without their bamboo."

"Scuppered?" queried Uncle.

"Yes, had it, bingo!" I said in explanation.

"This modern language!" sighed Uncle.

"Modern? That's what my mother says," I whispered under my breath.

"Well, our forerunners were more fortunate than those butterflies in that they found that there were several types of food that they could eat, including some plant foods.

But," continued Uncle Wolfi resolutely, "as the climate cooled and our forbears had to roam further and further afield, the landscape changed and they necessarily became ever more reliant on animal food.

For instance, up here, as I said before, they ate the reindeer, which ate the mosses and lichen. Perhaps there was no option," said Uncle glancing at the snow that lay all around us.

"Yes, I suppose they were luckier, Uncle," I replied uncomfortably, seeing his glance and thinking of the lack of plant food on the mountainside, of our game of the previous summer and of our imaginary supper by the lakeshore.

"And so it came about that, especially – but not only – in this part of the world, the balance tipped more and more in favour of eating animal food, sometimes exclusively."

"But it's disgusting, all this meat-eating," I broke out.

"Ah, there you have it. Instead of respecting our heritage, such a way of eating has become 'disgusting' and we think of our forerunners as savages who are best forgotten!"

"It's true," I agreed.

"Yes, Schatz, it's true."

So now I was Uncle's Schatz, his treasure, his little darling, not only his Spatz, his little Sparrow!

The path was broad and the snow, being crisp and firm, was quite a delight to walk, but time was getting on.

"Let us walk back," suggested Uncle Wolfi.

I was pleased, thinking he might then change the topic, but no such luck.

"Yet early man was far closer to us in kind than the apes we see in zoos. It is pre-man and early man – not the apes – who, over millions of years, paved the way for us.

During this long interval of time, many small but significant changes happened to make the bodies of our forerunners suited to the new way of eating.

Amongst other things, there were changes in their guts, changes in the way their insides could digest items of food, in their teeth, in their jawbones and in the shape of their skulls; importantly, their brains gradually grew bigger."

"You did say that there was always change along the way!" I nodded.

"This process proceeded very gradually. By two million years ago, tools were being used and . . ."

Here Uncle interrupted himself to explain:

"By that time, we are speaking of beings we broadly classify as 'man', yet who are still not quite 'Homo sapiens', the human beings that we are today.

We humans only became the modern type of people we are now roughly 120,000-100,000 years ago."

"Why does all this matter?" continued Uncle Wolfi. "The changes I just mentioned meant that, over that long period of time – those millions of years of pre-man and early man – the bodies of our predecessors were gradually but enduringly adapting themselves to a food intake made up, if not entirely then certainly predominantly, of animal food.

Note that these physical changes and also this adaptation to animal food had already happened by the time we first became who we are now."

Uncle Wolfi paused to make sure I was following. I don't think I was.

"We tend to overlook this part of our history, Sparrow. Yet perhaps – and this is a distinct possibility – the very fact that we ourselves came into existence as a unique species already fully adapted to a diet the mainstay of which was animal food is of vital significance.

Indeed, perhaps this holds a missing clue to our own wellbeing nowadays?

In fact, what if some of our current troubles . . . ?"

"What if?" I queried, wondering what was coming.

"Just what if," replied Uncle Wolfi with his droll smile.

6 RASPBERRIES

During term-time, I thought a lot about what I had heard that Easter. I went over it again and again in my mind. I longed for the summer holidays to come round so that Uncle and I could continue our discussion.

At last I was in Austria again. It was a hot afternoon and Uncle Wolfi and I were picking raspberries together in his large garden.

"But people didn't just hunt, did they!" I said, all of a sudden.

"No, I understand that they also scavenged any leftovers they could find, and they gathered shell fish, molluscs, termites and a lot of other small creatures, too," replied Uncle.

"What I mean, Uncle, is that people must have been eating plants thousands of years ago. You see I've just done a project on hunter/gatherers at school," I added in explanation.

"Yes, yes, of course, plant food will have been eaten now and then, depending on where and when people lived, on local conditions and on the changing climate.

Remember this was long before agriculture and in those days there were very few people – just small roaming bands – and a comparative plenty of animals for food.

It would also have been easier to gather, say, fruit in the tropics than in Northern Europe!"

"The hunting part, though, was important," emphasised Uncle Wolfi. "Didn't I read somewhere recently that even now the indigenous aborigines of Australia always prefer animal food if they can get it?"

"Kangaroos and sand lizards, beetles and grubs, rodents, birds, eggs – and even fish and sea cows, if they live near the coast", I said knowledgably but reluctantly, as this did not exactly support my case.

"Arguments as to the likely proportions of animal versus vegetable food are still going on at the moment.

My impression is that there are people who want to prove that the ancients ate more plant food than they probably did."

Did he mean me, I wondered? But no, it seemed not.

"Oh Sparrow, it does seem that some people are ashamed of our real ancestry, yet no other animal bows its head in shame when it follows its natural path. Imagine an abject eagle!"

I wanted to say something but Uncle Wolfi was wrapt in his own thoughts.

"Nowadays", he continued, "there is even talk of cereals as the natural and original food of man – not surprisingly, they are finding it quite difficult to prove!

And we must be wary of results that are trying to substantiate a belief system. Of course I understand modern sensibilities about such things . . ."

His voice tailed off and we continued picking raspberries in silence.

"Uncle," I said, calling him back to what I was trying to ask. "Gathering?"

"I am sorry, little Sparrow, you see it is such a big topic! Yes, the gathering of plant food.

Well, imagine you are a bushman trotting across a desert: you have failed to bag the giraffe that would have fed you and

40

your family for a week, wouldn't you relish any edible roots that you could grub up and cook? Of course you would! You are well exercised and you and your children are hungry, and those roots filled an aching void and carried you through to the next proper meal.

That situation is very different from wanting a bread roll round your hamburger, chips with your fish or pasta with your pizza, when you have already eaten twice that day, not to mention biscuits in between."

This last suggestion did not go down well with me.

"But I only eat biscuits when I am hungry," I protested.

"You, child, have never known real hunger," said Uncle, I thought a touch severely.

"Well, it sometimes feels like it!" I replied rather sulkily.

"Ah, yes, that can be a consequence of, shall we say, too much of a good thing," said Uncle Wolfi enigmatically. "But back to gathering. We already saw there wasn't much of a selection to be had round here.

However, we don't all live in the mountains of Austria, so what about round where you live in the North of England? What grows wild and is really sweet, would you say?"

"Honey!" I exclaimed.

"Technically honey is animal food and a rare luxury at that," remarked Uncle. "In terms of wild fruits, I admit a very ripe blackberry has a touch of sweetness, but have you ever tasted a wild damson or a raw crab apple?"

He had a point, had Uncle Wolfi. Raw haws were floury but not sweet, neither were wild strawberries, and I had tried raw elderberries and I had spat them out in disgust.

"Now think of the fruit and vegetables of today," continued Uncle. "The plants that still grow wild are probably more like those eaten by early nomadic humans.

Are these wild fruits and plants at all like the ones you get from the supermarket or greengrocer?"

"Oh, not at all, Uncle," I said thinking of all the sugar Mum had to put into her crab apple jelly, and remembering a very sweet orange I had recently enjoyed.

"You see, over the years, and especially recently, man has deliberately bred out the bitterness in plants and has changed fruit and vegetables to be ever sweeter – even Brussels sprouts and cabbages!"

"I read of 'even sweeter sweet corn' on a packet recently," I commented.

"Precisely!" said Uncle. "So one of the things to remember when you are putting your food together sensibly is just how different the fruit and vegetables of today are from the products of gathering in those olden days."

"They were not half so sweet" I agreed, "in fact not a quarter!" I reflected.

"And this is something these modern-day promoters of plant food eating would do well to remember," muttered Uncle.

"Come on! Let's take our own gathering in for tea," said Uncle brightening. "What say you to a bowl of raspberries with a good helping of whipped cream, topped with a few of those tiny almond macaroons your Aunt Helen bakes?"

"I say yummy, yummy, I'll have food in my tummy," I answered playfully.

"Perhaps, Sparrow, you would like to bring in some fresh dandelions and some plantain leaves to add to the salad for old time's sake? I know there are some down by the orchard. Afterwards, we will continue our most interesting chat."

"Oh, yes, Uncle, there's lots I want to know," I replied quite genuinely. But I wasn't sure about the dandelions!

After tea, we went for a walk.

"Oh, what a pretty little plant!" I exclaimed, crouching down to examine a mound of star-shaped leaves, outlined with silver, and stroking the soft silvery hairs on the underside of the leaves.

"Silbermänteli," said Uncle, "Little cloaks of silver."

"Silbermänteli," I repeated, "How lovely!"

"Lovely in a cup of tea, perhaps, though not in salad" said ever-practical Uncle. "Quite tough and hairy – that's part of the way such plants adapt themselves to the cold, and even so they go beneath the ground for the winter!"

"So we, as early humans, had animal food as the main part of our diet, with plant food when necessary and in season, and the plants were not always very filling and seldom very sweet," I summed up as best I could.

"Very good so far," said Uncle Wolfi. "Yes, as far as we know, that was our basic fare for something like a 100,000 years and, importantly, it is what our insides are organised to cope with – and efficiently, too."

"A hundred thousand years on meat and a few plants!" Now that was something to think about! Wow!

"And then came . . . ?" queried my relentless Uncle.

"Weetabix?" I ventured, "or maybe Cocopops?"

I pictured all those rows of colourful packets on the shelves of our local supermarket back home and even sighed a little at the recollection.

Seeing Uncle's frown, I rephrased my answer:

"Cereals? Wheat, barley, oats?"

"Yes, and then, of course, with cereals came bread."

"Bread, the staff of life," I responded, remembering the phrase from Sunday school.

"Not a staff I would care to lean on very heavily!" said Uncle dryly.

"Jesus broke bread with his disciples and they nibbled ears of corn," I remonstrated.

Stooping, Uncle Wolfi plucked a blade of wild grass and eyed it quizzically.

"Yes, that was roughly 2,000 years ago. To a youngster like you, that must sound a very long time but when you look at the history of mankind, it is very recent.

Of course, early humans, too, may have nibbled the odd grass seed or two but they did not, I think, eat bread."

"But Uncle, a hundred thousand years until we got bread!"

We walked on for a few minutes and then Uncle Wolfi resumed:

"What you probably don't realise, Schatz, is that, when we humans came onto the scene, the world was getting colder. In fact, it was just entering what we call the last Great Ice Age.

The coldest part was about 50,000 years ago. It then got slightly milder and the ice sheets advanced; they were at their most extensive about 18,000 years ago, whivch may seem strange but it is what I understand to have happened."

"And were sometimes incredibly thick!" I remembered.

"It was only after the ice started receding some 10-12,000 years ago that cereals entered the picture in any meaningful way. This was towards the end of this last Great Ice Age, when the climate was slowly warming again and the wild grasses we came to call cereals changed.

You see, it was only then – after this change – that we were able to grow them for food.

Since that time, over the millennia and especially recently, man has bred cereals into something very different from their original wild predecessors."

"I love cereals," I confessed.

Uncle ignored me:

"What is important is that cereals introduced a very different type of food into our diet.

Now, it is possible that our bodies have adapted a little to cereals over the past few thousand years, but in the big scheme of things, they are still a comparatively recent food."

"Oh Sparrow, just because we can eat both plants and animals, doesn't mean we can therefore eat indiscriminately each and every food we like.

Nor does it mean we can eat them in any quantity, of that I am sure," said Uncle with conviction.

"But Uncle . . ." I said, trying in vain to interrupt.

"You see, our bigger brains could solve bigger problems but I'm afraid we also created quite a few.

Perhaps domesticated and agricultural man thinks himself to be a new species? It is possible.

And by wrong thinking he justifies eating too much of the wrong type of food – food that then doesn't suit the workings of his body – and it makes him hungry for more of the same?"

"But, Uncle Wolfi, if you give a totally different type of food to a species unused to it – whose insides are expecting something else – what happens?"

"Trouble!" answered Uncle simply.

7 TROUBLE

"Uncle, can things go backward?" It was my first question
the next summer, as I had been wondering about this particular
question for a while. "For instance, if we chose to eat really
like apes do in the wild . . ."

"We would probably suffer a lot of gut ache!" rejoined
Uncle Wolfi with a smile.

"But lots of fruit and vegetables and a small amount of meat
and fat is a bit ape-like," I persisted.

"And there are a lot of gut problems around – in my line of
country, I should know!" countered Uncle.

"Oh, Uncle, I'm trying to ask you a serious question. On
such a diet, would our brains grow smaller again?"

"A very fair question!" answered Uncle Wolfi laughing.
"It's not absolutely impossible, though naturally it could take a
good few million years!"

I was beginning to feel offended at his laughter when he
paused and said:

"Well, done! You really have been doing some thinking!
Your question does raise the larger question as to how far our
basic diet is an integral part of our humanity, of our uniqueness
as human beings."

Here Uncle Wolfi drew a long breath. At the time, we were
walking together in his large garden. Uncle stopped and held
out his hands to help me up onto a large tree stump so that I
had a better view of the lake.

"What? Such cold hands you have, little one, and in summer,
too. Are they always like that?" he queried and I nodded.

"And sometimes my feet are absolutely freezing!"

"Hmm!" was his only comment. "Na ja, jump down and we'll walk round to the orchard and sit on the wall. There's so much to untangle, like when a kitten has been playing with the knitting wool!"

I put my cold hand not into his hand but in his arm to show I was getting older. I was twelve and was now at secondary school.

As we walked, I imagined this tall old man beside me was leading me into a giant maze – there had been so much talk and arguing at school about diet. Yet, walking with Uncle, I felt content and somehow trusting.

Anyway, we wouldn't get lost because Uncle Wolfi was so tall he could probably see over the hedges!

"Where do I begin?" he asked.

"You could try with trouble," I suggested.

"Yes, trouble!" Uncle sighed wistfully. "Trouble comes, but not always immediately, sometimes not for a long time . . .

Our bodies are quite amazing and bend over backwards to do all they can to keep us well: make do, compensate for our errors, bring in a whole host of balancing and emergency measures and so on.

However, there is a cost to all this constant adjusting and compensating and, sooner or later, the consequences of this indulgence, or maybe we should say the consequences of this misguided practice, catch up with us."

Uncle was losing me fast and, noticing this, he changed his approach:

"Now, remember you told me of how, every day for weeks, your neighbour was feeding a blackbird raisins, how it was not long before that bird came tapping on the window with its beak for more and how your neighbour was delighted the blackbird had made such friends with her.

Well, yes, she did feel befriended by the bird but really it was coming for its regular fix. It is like, like . . ."

"Like me going to the sweet shop on my way home from school?" I ventured.

"And for the same reasons," rejoined Uncle, nodding his head sagely. "Not good, not good! So much concentrated sweetness is unnatural for a blackbird and it unbalances the bird's system.

Did you notice anything else about the blackbird?"

"Well, I know there were three nests built that year rather than the usual one or two."

"Interesting," commented Uncle.

Here Uncle Wolfi got up from the hard stone wall on which we were sitting and had a stretch. We then walked together at a leisurely pace through the old fruit trees.

"And it is not just sweetness that does it, you know."

Then somewhat unexpectedly, he added:

"Take hens: I did an experiment once – and without the temptation of raisins!"

"Not a nasty animal experiment, Uncle?" I said, immediately on my guard.

"If you call 'nasty' giving my chickens something like their original diet, I plead guilty. Naturally, I couldn't give them the grubs and insects they might have had in a Borneo rainforest, but I gave them shrimps and other such delicacies."

"And what happened, Uncle?"

"In short, my birds were much healthier and had lovely plumage, whereas the others that were fed on their normal cereal feed – and which came running for more – got their normal troubles."

"Is that why you don't eat cornflakes for breakfast?"

"So that I grow shiny feathers, you mean?" said Uncle, stroking the thinning white hair on the top of his head.

Uncle was exasperating at times!

"But guess what happened to the egg production of my superb birds," chuckled Uncle.

"They had lots and lots of beautiful eggs that were even bigger and there were even more of them," I suggested.

"Quite the reverse: the eggs were smaller and there were hardly any of them – in no time, the hens laid just two lots of eggs a year, behaving like the wild birds they once were!"

"But I thought chickens just laid masses of eggs naturally and that's why people like keeping them," I said in surprise, for this was a lot to take in.

"Not at all! Chickens are ordinary birds," explained Uncle Wolfi. "They have been long domesticated by us, it is true, but they only produce an abnormally large number of eggs if aided and abetted by us in the way we feed them.

Ask any farmer's wife why she feeds chickens corn! She'll tell you it is to get them to lay."

I thought about this for a while. Still puzzled I asked:

"Uncle, are you saying that it is the cereal that makes chickens lay so many eggs and for months on end? But why? How can that be?"

"It seems that, given in quantity, cereal – or rather what cereal contains – somehow disturbs the bird's reproductive system."

Now, that had never occurred to me: how could it?

"Oh heavens! I hope it doesn't do that to us!" I exclaimed, alarmed at my own thought.

"Now you really are beginning to put the right questions, my young chickaboo!

Unfortunately, there are many ways in which this can disturb us, too, ways you will no doubt learn about as you get older."

Uncle Wolfi noticed my anxious face and softened slightly:

"Don't be frightened, Sparrow. After all, when we removed the cereal from my birds' feed, their reproductive systems did normalise. It is just something worth thinking about.

Perhaps a food, which is useful as a reserve to fall back on in lean times, can become harmful when it becomes a staple food, especially an over-plentiful one?

What do you think?" As I made no reply, he added:

"Rest assured, we do have a choice in the matter."

Uncle Wolfi now sat down on a wooden bench, patting the place next to him and I sat too.

"When you feed an animal – or a human for that matter – with a type of food that does not belong to its natural past, there are so many things that can, and do, go wrong, some of which you wouldn't ever think were food-related.

I have found that disturbances express themselves in so many ways . . ."

"Oh Uncle Wolfi, must you?" I pleaded, but he carried on.

"Now our forefathers were programmed for a frugal and sometimes intermittent food intake, with the occasional, hmm, binge?" he said, looking at me to check he had got the right modern word.

"Binge is right," I acknowledged.

"If we ourselves no longer eat this way, but tend not just to eat very frequently but to eat quite a quantity of food, too, then you can see that a constant 'too much' might constitute quite a problem of overload.

And if, into the bargain, this constant 'too much' consists of an unexpected type of food, there you have it!

In other words, it's not just all feast and no famine, but these days, it is the wrong sort of feast to start with!"

I was close to tears. It was all too much.

"But we don't want to talk about all this now, do we, Spatz? Surely, the good thing to hold in our minds is that it is possible to eat in a way that makes trouble less likely and, moreover, which brings all sorts of benefits in all sorts of unexpected ways," said Uncle, smiling reassuringly.

"And our little cell engines?" I asked, not quite reassured, and remembering our time together in the boat three summers before.

"As you can imagine, these function most effectively on their primary fuel and they 'burn' it cleanly."

"So all would then be OK?" I asked.

"Well, with other fuel, the little engines have to work twice as hard for the same output, and there can be waste that is not always easily got rid of and can clog things up.

You see, if there is too much of the less welcome fuel, some of it gets processed not in the little engines but in the spaces inside the cell and processed without oxygen.

I should mention that all parts of the body don't have the same preference for fuel, but these miniature powerhouses sort this all out among themselves very well, that is as long as the overall supply of food from outside is in more or less the right quantity and the right mix.

51

There is a lot of leeway, but too much of the wrong thing and there does come a time . . ."

Poor Uncle Wolfi, he did keep veering back to the thought of ailments and once he got going there was no stopping him. But then he was a doctor and how to get people well again had been the focus of his life's work.

"There might come a time . . . well, I have this hunch that if the fuel mix sent to the cells to process is too unlike what our cells hope for to function normally . . . then there will be too much fermenting going on and not enough oxygen around and, well, it is just possible that at least some of our trillions of cells will think they are again living in the primordial soup and act accordingly."

What planet does Uncle live on! I looked at him now as uncomprehendingly as I had when he first mentioned this strange soup.

"And then . . ." he finished, throwing up his hands in a bleak gesture of impending doom.

Suddenly his eyes twinkled:

"Do you believe me when I tell you all these things, some of which I admit are very unusual?"

"I try to, Uncle Wolfi, that is I do when I think you're not joking!" I said timidly.

"Believe it or not, I am not asking you to accept what I say. Yes, there are some things for which we have to take the word of others, but we can still do our own thinking.

Never forget that! As I have found myself, things become more meaningful when you discover them for yourself."

"When I first started thinking about the way we eat," Uncle reflected, "I doubted it all myself!

52

I very much needed to prove to myself that I was on the right lines, so I tried my ideas out on myself just to see.

In fact, for four years I didn't have any cereal at all and not many sweet things either."

"Sounds awful," I said, imaging life without bread, jam or breakfast cereal.

"Actually, it wasn't so bad at all," said Uncle, reminiscing.

"What happened?" I asked curiously.

"I was calmer, had less aches and pains, and was fitter. In fact, it turned me round and I had a whole new lease of life."

"Really, Uncle?"

"Oh yes, but perhaps what I did in those first four years was a bit extreme. I eased up a little after that. That was over forty years ago and for me it has been very liberating.

Yes, very liberating for it is not as though I can't eat and drink whatever I like, I can – and you know my penchant for gourmet foods!

It's just that I choose to be very modest in the portion sizes of certain foods, that's all."

"That's all," I repeated, smiling at Uncle's understatement.

"Come on, it is getting late. Let us go in for our supper. I think you will find that the real proof of the eating is in one of your Aunt Helen's scumptious, if somewhat tiny, puddings!"

"Scrumptious," I corrected, glad of the chance to do so, but looking forward to the pudding nonetheless.

8 BLUE IRISES

I was sitting on the doorstep with my head in my hands, deeply puzzled, when Uncle came by. He stopped and looked at me enquiringly.

"I have a problem, Uncle Wolfi," I admitted.

"Can I help, little one?" Uncle still sometimes called me this.

"I have found what you say fascinating and honestly it makes a lot of sense, it's just that . . ." I faltered.

"Go on," said Uncle gently.

"Well, it's just that I'm worried by the fact that it is precisely those things which must have been central to our original diet as humans that our teachers say are bad for us. They are going to be given red traffic lights!" I blurted out.

It was Uncle Wolfi's turn to look puzzled. He nodded toward the garden and I followed slowly.

"What is it, Schatz? Is there something in particular that's troubling you?"

"Fat!"

"Fat?" echoed Uncle Wolfi.

"Yes, fat," I grunted. "Well, meat and fat but mainly fat."

"Go on," said Uncle gently. I grunted some more. "Come on, let's go to our favourite bench under the apple trees."

We walked in silence, surrounded by bird song and looking at the wild flowers peeping out of the grass.

"My teacher says . . ." I began when we reached the bench, but I was interrupted.

"Hush, hush," said Uncle. He has a way of saying words twice. "I know that at school they tell you that fat is a problem

54

food, especially animal fat, and that you should eat very little of it or it will make you ill.

But let me ask you something: have you ever got 'the wrong end of the stick'? Have you ever cheated a little bit to win an argument? For example, have you ever been too clever? Have you ever 'proved' something in such a way that you have left common sense behind and ended up, well, with a result that is quite ridiculous, even absurd?"

"Oh dear, yes!" I confessed, still gruff.

"Of course you have – and probably enjoyed it, too!" Here I had to smile for I knew it was true.

Uncle paused, folding his arms.

"Well, that's what has happened with the people who have dreamt up what we call the 'fat theory': namely the theory that fats traditional to our tables are harmful to us. Some adults have cheated a little, some have been too clever, others have been duped, whilst still others have thought of a way of making lots of money out of the myth-making.

For you, pretence when arguing and joking is just fun but this, shall we say misinterpretation by adults, deliberate or not, is serious as it has led to a great many people being made ill."

"With nasty horrid diseases!"

"With severe afflictions certainly.

It has also led to a lot of people struggling to get well whilst following advice which all the time is making them ill, which you must admit is quite absurd!"

"Take all those studies one keeps hearing about. Often they claim to prove something after trying a diet for only a fortnight, or else they begin from the wrong starting point because the established so-called 'facts' aren't questioned, yet ought to be.

55

Best to deal with the conclusions of such studies by holding them all very lightly. And never just read the conclusions – they can be very misleading – always read the middle as well and you'll see how some of this absurdity came about!"

Uncle was climbing on his hobbyhorse. I enjoyed watching him, all fired up.

"Never, in the whole history of man, I tell you, has such an unnatural diet been put forward with such determination, with such expense and with such spurious scientific grounding!"

Seeing the expression on my face, Uncle stopped abruptly.

"Oh Sparrow, if you only knew how we have been misled into believing the myths about fat. And how much harm this has done!

Moreover, people have been made too afraid to trust the wisdom of their own bodies. They are taught not only to despise tradition but also the food of their own grandparents, even if their own grandparents were comparatively healthy.

Soon enough I will give you lots of learned books so that you can study and judge all the nonsense for yourself.

For now, one word suffices: RIDICULOUS!"

"We were talking just now of animal food as an integral part of the diet of humankind, well yes, it has been so for more than a 100,000 years: that is for as long as mankind has existed," confirmed Uncle.

"This means that both the fat and the lean of meat were foodstuffs so fundamental to our diet that we, as humans, owed our very existence to them!" he continued.

"Food so ancient that it was once our only food," I put in.

"Yes, Spatz, always keep a long enough view of history! And keep on asking one particular question," urged Uncle.

"That being?" I asked.

"The question being: how could such foodstuffs so long in our diet in themselves suddenly become so bad for us?"

"HOW COULD FOODSTUFFS THAT HAVE BEEN SO VERY LONG IN OUR DIET SUDDENLY BECOME BAD FOR US?" I repeated with emphasis, echoing his equally loud 'ridiculous' and tapping my head with each word to help me remember it. "Such ancient foods all of a sudden becoming so harmful to us humans? It doesn't make sense," I concurred.

"Good old Sparrow, you really are getting my point!"
I felt a glow of warmth at Uncle Wolfi's approval.

Later, we strolled down to the rose bed together. After a while, Uncle said quietly:

"The tide of thought has not yet turned, particularly amongst the high-ups, and the old guidelines are still in place.

In the prevailing climate of opinion, such a way of eating as I propose is only thought well of by those who practise it and so know its worth.

It is a difficult one. I stuck my neck out and I know the cost from my own experience."

"I stick my neck out every time I speak up in class," I complained.

"And your teachers don't say the same as I do?"
Had Uncle read my mind?

"This is why, for the time being, my advice to you is to store this question inwardly."

Uncle had a faraway look as if recalling distant happenings.

"My colleagues – those that are sympathetic to my work, that is – handle the problem very delicately.

They don't advertise the fact that they use my diet in their treatment of certain ailments, but practise its principles discreetly both on themselves and on a one-to-one basis with patients," he remarked, as if to himself.

Uncle paused, correcting himself:

"I know I should not call it 'my' diet, and you know that, too," he added, I thought almost humbly. "And people can be so impetuous – I tended to be so myself – and too much haste can bring problems.

One-to-one is the safest way. Yes, best not to shout it from the rooftops, even though you might feel like doing so at times, best not even to argue about it."

"No arguing!" I repeated dutifully.

"I had hoped the tide would turn in my lifetime, but I doubt that it will. Na ja, na ja!" muttered Uncle Wolfi, with an expression half sad, half amused on his face.

Perhaps he was thinking of 'all those studies'?

"Look at the colour of those roses! Isn't it wonderful?"

"Heavenly," I said, bending to smell them. "Hmm, perfect!"

"You see, the emphasis of our diet may have changed recently – or rather the official script may have changed – but the question here is this: has the construction and organisation of our bodies changed sufficiently in the meantime to make our long-term foods harmful? Surely not!

Watch, listen, read round the subject, learn what you can. Above all, as I said, keep your own counsel and your ability to think for yourself."

"Thank you, Uncle, I'll remember your advice."

Uncle Wolfi stooped to dead-head one of his roses.

"It's all very simple really: things work better when we are what we are, and are not trying to be something else!" said he.

I grinned: that bit was a riddle no longer.

"To be healthy," mused Uncle, "yes, I know atmospheric and other types of pollution have to be dealt with, as well as other issues such as insufficient exercise and unwholesome surroundings. I am well aware of all that.

In terms of nutrition, in my view, there is one basic rule: that we have to learn to eat and drink in a way which, as far as possible, keeps the workings of our body comfortably within the normal boundaries of the body's internal operating system.

Overload is anything that unduly disturbs this working balance – and my colleagues know well how one imbalance leads to another!" he said, falling back into his own thoughts.

Eating and drinking in a way that suits our operating system – such an old man using computer speak!

I was impressed, but I was none the wiser. Uncle Wolfi had said similar things many times, yet I still could make neither head nor tail of it. All this talk of being 'designed' in a certain way meant nothing to me.

Then I realised that, apart from the snippets I had learnt from Uncle, I hadn't the faintest idea about how my body worked or even how it was supposed to work when it functioned well.

No wonder I couldn't understand much of what Uncle was saying to me.

I shook my head despondently:

"I'm not sure I quite understand you, Uncle."

"In time, you can learn all about it, Sparrow," said Uncle Wolfi comfortingly, "and maybe there will come a time when you will want to do your own little experiment and try out my way of eating for yourself. If so, I'm happy to be your guide."

That evening, I still felt a niggle in the back of my mind. What Uncle said was so, so different from what my teachers said, even though I was now at senior school.

It must have showed on my face during our evening meal, because Uncle raised one eyebrow in my direction and went on eating his roast pork.

At the end of the first course, Uncle Wolfi wiped his mouth with his napkin, folded it carefully and then beckoned me with one finger to come with him.

Feeling both uncomfortable and curious, I followed him into his study.

"Now stand right over here with me and look at the picture on the far wall. What do you see?" he asked.

"Flowers," I said, "I think they're blue irises."

"Now go up very closely to them and have another look," said Uncle.

"Great splodges of paint!" I said laughing, "and I thought Monet was a great artist!"

"Perhaps he still is," replied Uncle Wolfi with a twinkle.

Walking to the window, he turned a thoughtful look on me.

"Perhaps our knowledge of history – and of nutrition – is a bit like a painting: not exactly great splodges of paint, as you so charmingly put it, but certainly a brushstroke here, a flick of paint there.

The trouble is that people argue with one blurred dash of colour against another, and especially when it comes to arguments about what to eat.

Little Sparrow, we all have a tendency to draw conclusions from little splashes, as though they were exact details and not just a tiny part of the picture. It can be very confusing and I confess I am no exception. There is still a lot we don't know.

As for my part, I am an old man and it is now up to others to fill in some of the finer details of my own larger canvas. My

60

hope is that by enough people standing far enough back, the real picture will come into focus."

"I like that idea," said I.

"I am fairly sure I have got the broad outlines correct. Yes, I think my bigger picture will stand up to the test, and that scientific research will prove me right in time.

Did you know that there is a long tradition of using art to illustrate science? The ancient Chinese were particularly good at it," he concluded with a smile.

I hugged him appreciatively, but Uncle Wolfi held me at arm's length and looked me in the eyes.

"My advice to you about what to eat is to stay very modest with your intake of recent foods – and you know by now what I mean by recent – and then your own body will soon be your guide. It will tell you when it is happy or when you are overstepping the mark."

"Will it?" I asked, looking up at him gratefully.

"It will do, if you learn to listen to it properly, that is," answered Uncle Wolfi. "Does it not remind you with that over-filled feeling when you have over-indulged, to give a small example."

"When I've pigged myself, you mean?

"That is one way of putting it, I suppose," said Uncle. "I would prefer to say when you have eaten too much."

"Treasure what I have told you in your heart, as I said," continued Uncle with a reassuring smile, "and share it only when you feel it might help someone.

Who knows, later on the time may come when you, little Sparrow, will tell my story."

I looked surprised but Uncle Wolfi at last returned my hug.

"Come on, let's go and finish our supper," he said, offering his arm and leading the way.

Next day, I was down by the pond inventing a game in which Uncle Wolfi was a wizened old wizard with a long flowing beard and healing people with his wand. Then I remembered his objection to magic and started adapting a poem I knew:

> You are old, Uncle Wolfi, the young girl said,
> And your hair has become very white,
> And yet you incessantly stand on your head –
> Do you think, at your age, it is right?

Uncle surprised me.

"What am I standing on its head now, little one?" he asked, mishearing me.

"Oh, I have just been going over in my mind some of the discussions I have had with you, Uncle, over the last few years," I replied, which was true.

"For instance, all that you once said about us coming out of what went before, but there always being change along the way," I said balancing on tip-toe along the stones at the edge of the pond.

"Funny you should say that, Sparrow, as at the moment I'm working on a new theory.

Salt is very important to our bodies and the way they work. Well, I have been studying the history of our relationship to salt from the very earliest days: that is from the time of the single-celled organism onwards.

In fact, I've been inspired by coelacanths. No, there are none in this pond," he said, following the direction of my eyes, "they lived millions of years ago."

"Salt and old fish?" I said, ceasing my game and screwing up my face in puzzlement.

"Yes, Sparrow, salt and old fish!" said Uncle laughing, "but just don't you worry your little head about the fanciful notions of an old man!"

"Uncle, you are quite amazing!" I exclaimed delighted, for to me my white-haired Uncle was not old but already ancient.

"No, no, child," he said modestly, "I am not amazing at all. I merely apply lessons that I have learnt from history, lessons which are there for all of us to learn."

"Oh, you are not any old man, Uncle Wolfi," I protested, "you are the old man from the mountains of Austria – the old man, who has a priceless secret because he is so old that he remembers things other people forgot!"

PART II

WONDERING

9 WHAT IF?

After that last memorable scene by the pond, I only saw Uncle Wolfi twice. In my teens, I was ever busy with schooling and exams. Uncle, too, though in his eighties, was still busy with his medical work.

Those enchanting summer holidays spent with him at his home in Austria became a thing of the past. My recollections of those earlier times mostly dwindled into fantasy, yet our fascinating conversations remained vivid.

After my last visit, Uncle Wolfi and Aunt Helen adopted a pattern of annual migration, spending their winters in England and their summers in Austria.

The large house of my dreams was sold. That must have been a sad day, for I remember Uncle Wolfi telling me proudly how he had designed it himself. Now, the house had been pulled down by someone wishing to build an even bigger one and not a trace of the house or garden remains.

Though we saw each other seldom, Uncle Wolfi kept in touch with his 'little Sparrow' – for he still used this quaint endearment that he had used for me as a child.

I had been so intrigued by what he had told me about his journey of discovery that it had set me off on my own journey. I studied a lot, reading anything that I could find that seemed relevant. Uncle and I discussed, argued and at times almost fought over ideas.

Bit by bit, with Uncle Wolfi's help, I began piecing things together. During our voluminous correspondence and phone calls, I was to have many chances to ask Uncle questions. Over time, he was to send me copies of his various German books.

And still I puzzled on.

Uncle Wolfi liked to think that he had inherited an inventive streak from his great-grandfather, who had constructed a very successful automated mill, powered by the rushing waters of the river Ache as it tumbled its way through the Tyrol.

Before Uncle became a doctor, he had been a medical scientist. I remember him telling me all about how he had designed a prototype of the modern space suit. He also told me of the engines he himself had designed and that he had patents of some of them pending. I had great respect for Uncle Wolfi as an inventor.

Uncle's father had been a village doctor in Upper Austria, and he, too, had possessed a practical streak. During the school holidays, 'young Wolfi' would often accompany his father on his rounds to outlying farms. In wintertime, they would go together on skis.

On these visits, he witnessed how his father not only treated the various ailments of his patients but would also willingly turn his hand to whatever was necessary.

What it must have been like watching his dad extract teeth or minister to their sick cows!

When Uncle Wolfi became a physician himself, it was as a problem-solver that he turned his attention to the seemingly ever-increasing incidence of serious disease.

The shortest letter that I ever received from Uncle Wolfi contained just two words: 'What if?'

It was a frequent phrase of his, but that letter was especially delightful because, to me, it summed him up.

Yes, Uncle W was a 'what if' man: a practical, problem-solving man who asked 'what if things don't work quite like that', or 'what if we have got it wrong', or 'what if we try such and such a way instead and see if it works'?

Uncle seemed to apply this 'what if' approach to theories as well as to everyday medicine. Yet he was not a random trial and error man: rather he was thoughtful and always looking for the reasons why things happened as they did.

In my earliest memories, Uncle was already an old man. By then, Uncle Wolfi had found a few answers – and very challenging ones they were, too!

So perhaps it was inevitable that I, in my turn, was led to ask 'what if', and even to put to myself the most daunting question of all:

WHAT IF UNCLE WOLFI WAS RIGHT?

- right in his view of evolutionary history
- right about our ancient diet being mainly of animal food
- right about being tuned to frugality and periods of want
- right about the link between what we ate and the inner workings of our bodies
- right about us not exactly being designed for stacks of cake and biscuits?

OH, HEAVEN FORBID!

10   BARBARIC YAWP

I was in my early teens when I began to explore the ideas of Uncle Wolfi for myself.

First of all, I needed to find the 'time before bread' that Uncle had talked about, so I started looking into our distant past. I got so excited about what I read that I rang Uncle Wolfi, who was in London at the time.

"Uncle, guess what? I've found tough and hairy hominids, ape-men and tree-men and other ever less hairy but not quite men. In fact, I've found what amounts to a whole family tree of our early ancestors."

"No, Sparrow, it was not a family tree: it was a bush!" he remonstrated.

"I can't talk about a family bush!" I protested.

"There were a lot of different stems as well as branches," he countered.

"A bush-like family tree, then? But, oh, how long it took each group to change into something else!"

"Yes, Sparrow, a long slow journey to mankind over many millions of years."

I could almost see Uncle Wolfi nodding into the phone.

"Yes, Uncle," I agreed enthusiastically. "Then came Homo this and Homo that, Homos with all sorts of long complicated names and, eventually, came Homo sapiens – that's us!"

I was learning Latin at school, so I knew by now that Homo sapiens meant 'knowing man'. I felt this to be a bit arrogant on our part: after all, our predecessors had known fire for, some say, two million years before we came on the scene. And who is to say they did not barbecue their steaks like we do now?

Uncle had told me that the last lot had bigger brains than us; I read that they also had tools, wore primitive clothing and they could make shelters like our own early kin.

Maybe these skills had passed from one developing group to another? In the books I consulted, it didn't say. Evidence as to their lives seemed to come from the odd pile of very old bones and occasionally a complete skeleton with a few fragments of animal remains from the same cave.

Nevertheless, it was widely held that those before us were a pretty carnivorous bunch.

From all accounts, we 'Homo sapiens' were also a pretty carnivorous bunch! This I knew in theory, as Uncle was always going on about it.

What really surprised me was the level of agreement among the experts on the subject, not only as to the predominance of meat in our diet over that long period of time but also as to its excellence as a form of nutrition.

Time and again I found mention of the superb physique, tall stature, strength and health of early Homo sapiens, which they had no hesitation in attributing to their 'excellent all-meat diet'.

Yet, in the past, Mum had made me feel guilty if I relished a piece of pork scratching that was to be given only to the dog!

Something did not add up.

"Uncle," I said to Uncle Wolfi on another occasion, "as far as I can see, the experts all seem to think that our ancient diet made people really fit and well.

I wonder what those experts eat for their own dinner? Do they try to follow the example of our ancestors or do they eat beans on toast like the rest of us?"

70

Uncle Wolfi chuckled:

"I very much doubt that they want to emulate those whom they feel to be savages! Though I think some of us still have some sort of primaeval yearning for at least some animal food in our diet."

"I myself like a good Bolognese but not without the spaghetti," I put in.

"And don't you think it is possible that our genes remember that distant past?" he continued.

"Could be," said I.

"I saw a lovely story in one of your English newspapers. London businessmen were reported queuing to buy pork pies after work to eat on the way home in order to fill in advance the gap in the low fat, meatless meal they knew they would face that evening!" and still chuckling, Uncle rang off.

My next port of call was Uncle Wolfi's hero: the explorer Vilhjalmur Stefansson, known familiarly as Stef. Uncle said this was the closest I would be able to get to meeting our Ice-Age relatives.

I therefore borrowed 'My Life with the Eskimo' from our local library and I soon trudged, slid and sledged with Stef across the Arctic.

On my travels, I met traditional Inuit families called Copper Eskimos, who had never previously met a white man – this was at the beginning of the 20th century – and, oh dear, they really did live off animal food and happily, too, it seems.

Further confirmation of an unpalatable fact!

However, the Inuit seemed far from savage: from what I read, they were welcoming, polite and considerate to visitors like Stef and his companion. It may, of course, have helped that Stef already spoke their language.

I began to feel a growing respect for these supposedly primitive people. They fed and clothed their children, were kind enough to take food to other families in the group who had a shortage, kept dogs, made sleds, made needles to sew their own clothes and made their own copper knives with which to prepare food.

They knew, too, how to ventilate their snow houses, which they heated with oil lamps, and enjoyed singing and dancing during the long dark winter days.

Just imagine sub-zero temperatures outside and a whole family living in one room – and a room with walls of snow, lined with ice. They slept, not on beds as we know them, but on platforms made of ice and covered with animal furs.

Yet they were able not only to keep the place warm but to cook and dry their clothes and boots with just one lamp that used whale or seal oil. Amazing!

Moreover, the inside temperature of their snow houses apparently kept at 21 – 26 degrees Celsius while the cooking was going on and the igloo subsequently kept warm all night.

Our house in northern England never got as warm as 26°!

One surprise was that, if sufficient food was to hand, these Inuit families chose to eat three meals a day just like we do – only with us it is three main meals plus snacks.

Yes, and cook these people did. They tossed lean caribou meat into molten ice that had been brought to the boil, cooked it just enough to suit their taste and then ate the boiled meat together with cold uncooked fat.

For afters, they drank the cooking water. Perhaps they, too, liked a nice hot drink, a bit like us with our cups of tea?

So when things went well, the particular Inuit I was reading about had warm houses and cooked meals, let alone sung and danced. It all sounded very civilised!

However, when I tried to equate seal flipper for breakfast with the sausage and tomato I used to enjoy at Uncle Wolfi's as a child, my imagination failed me miserably.

It was probably just me, though, for I later read how, on one expedition, Stefansson instructed his men to 'go native'; some were reluctant at first but, with eating just seal meat, none took more than two weeks at the most to feel comfortable and well.

All in all, Stefansson found a robust and helpful community. Life for the Inuit was not all roses: not that there were any roses, but there were flowers on the tundra in summertime!

I talked to my classmates about all this. They said the Inuit were only healthy because they ate all their food raw – and ate mostly fish at that.

I thought about what Stefansson had said to the contrary. Stef spent very many years in the Arctic and he found that some Inuit ate fish, others ate meat such as musk ox or seal, whilst some ate both meat and fish, depending on availability.

And yes, sometimes they would eat their fish or meat raw in an almost frozen state but it seems that, like the Copper Eskimos, they mostly cooked it.

My classmates also said the Inuit ate berries and that was how they got their vitamins and that without these they could not have lived. I thought how berries were only available very occasionally and just at the end of their short summer.

I replied that maybe the gathering of the Inuit was almost entirely of the animal kind. This suggestion did not go down well. In fact, I was not at all believed and I began to understand why Uncle Wolfi had advised me to say little.

So I just muttered inwardly 'berries, my foot!'

I found further evidence that it was not berries that kept the old-style Inuit healthy, when I read another of Stef's books called The Friendly Arctic.

On an expedition across the ice, Stef was joined by three men who had ignored his advice to include fresh meat in their daily fare and who had been secretly living off store groceries for the previous few months.

The men got ill and steadily worsened; it turned out they had developed scurvy. I had read somewhere that scurvy comes from not having enough vitamin C, so obviously fruit, and especially oranges and lemons, was necessary.

Yet after returning to land, all three men were subsequently cured, not by being given fruit and veg – for there weren't any available – but with lightly boiled fresh fat caribou meat. This they were given for breakfast and, only if they needed further meals during the day, were they given the meat raw.

In two to three days, their depression had lifted, in two weeks they could walk ten miles and in just a month were apparently restored to full health.

All this got me thinking, for this had to mean that it was not just oranges that contained vitamin C. I knew that sailors took sauerkraut on long sea voyages but sauerkraut was made from cabbages, so that didn't count.

Then I remembered that Captain Cook took live animals such as sheep and hens along with him to provide fresh meat for his men and Captain Cook's sailors didn't get scurvy.

I told my classmates about the scurvy. We searched on the wall charts at school, but meat was not listed under vitamin C on any of them. So my classmates still didn't believe it was possible to be in good health just eating meat.

Hold it lightly, Sparrow, hold it lightly! I must speak to Uncle Wolfi about all this, too.

So I again phoned Uncle, who laughed:

"Well you know, you are not alone. Vilhjalmur Stefansson himself was not believed!"

"Surely not!" I exclaimed, a little shocked.

"Oh yes. But then we Westerners often find such things difficult to believe. Maybe we have drifted too far from our forefathers?"

"But what about the vitamin C, Uncle?"

"Ah, for any animal, when it comes to an essential need such as for vitamin C, there are only two options: either it can be eaten or the body itself can manufacture it."

"Well, fresh fat meat did cure scurvy!"

"There you have it!" said Uncle in his enigmatic way.

"Now, Stefansson wrote many books and articles about what he had observed in the Arctic. His word was doubted, as I said, especially when it came to the scurvy bit and how he and his men were living happily on meat alone.

In fact, in the late 1920's, several doctors were so sceptical about white men being able to live on meat alone – the Inuit were different, they said – that an experiment was set up in a New York hospital. Let me tell you about it," said Uncle.

"Oh please do. I know you had to do an experiment even just to prove your diet to yourself."

"And therefore I know first-hand that there's nothing so convincing as direct experience!

Anyway, this is how things went: after an initial medical check-up, Stef was given lean meat only. This was despite his protest for, in the Arctic, he had seen with his own eyes the devastation caused by lack of fat in a diet. I remember he called such a diet a rabbit diet . . ."

"Sorry?" I said, not following.

"Rabbits don't have much fat on them," explained Uncle Wolfi, "and when the Inuit only had lean meat to eat they got terribly ill. Of course, they couldn't eat just fat either. To be healthy, they needed some of each, both the fat and the lean."

"I don't think I could eat butter without the toast", I put in with feeling, "or cream without the apple pie."

"As I was saying, at first Stef was allowed to eat only lean meat and, in just two days, it had made him unwell."

"Bunged him up?" I suggested.

"Not at all," replied Uncle.

"Gave him the trots?" I guessed.

"Correct, whereas his former companion of the Copper Eskimo days, who was put straight onto meat with the fat on, had no such trouble. Once fat was allowed, Stef was soon well again. That surprises you, doesn't it!"

"A little," I admitted.

"Well, both of them then spent a whole year eating just fresh fat meat – note not organic meat or wild game, just ordinary butcher's meat – and with a free choice as to which meat and the amount of fat and lean."

"A whole year! Unbelievable!"

"Yes, a whole year. They were allowed to eat and cook their meat in any way they chose: grilled, roasted, braised or boiled Inuit style; black coffee was also allowed.

The men chose mostly to cook their meat: his companion liked it medium, whilst Stef preferred it well done."

I held my breath in suspense as Uncle paused. "And what happened?" I asked eagerly.

"The doctors, professors and nutritionists stood around and watched, expecting them both to drop dead at any moment!

Well, they didn't exactly stand round: they measured every single thing they could measure and were unbelievably thorough with all their examinations.

Interestingly, a gut specialist made the comment that, had he been consulted, he would have advised Stef's companion that in order to cure his gut problems he should refrain from eating any meat at all."

"And, Uncle, and?"

"Result: not a single sign of scurvy and not a single raising or lowering of any indicator that pointed to any worsening of their health.

Stef, who was well at the start of the experiment, stayed well and – ironically – his companion who, as an orange farmer in Florida, had had a few previous problems, especially with his gut, became well."

What can one say? To think of two men living in a big city being healthy eating just ordinary fat meat and no other food!

Didn't it suggest that meat really was a complete food that provided everything that was needed? It had to, surely?

And now the experts were confirming that, with animal food as the main and sometimes sole item of their diet, our early relatives were supremely healthy.

So what Uncle Wolfi had told me was all too horribly true?

A little passage came to mind from Walt Whitman's long poem
Song of Myself:

> The spotted hawk swoops by . . .
> I too am not a bit tamed, I too am untranslatable,
> I sound my barbaric yawp over the roofs of the world.

Uncle Wolfi certainly had a 'barbaric yawp': writing as he
did of our kinship with 'savages', who ate little else but the
flesh and fat of animals.

And this our rightful heritage? Ugh!

Uncle had said as much during my holidays in Austria, but I
suppose I hoped he had been exaggerating!

And how strange that such a sophisticated person with no
coarseness, roughness or barbarism about him – and such a
lover of good food, too – should see such a barbaric way of
eating as the blueprint for health!

It is not as though he, himself, lived on just meat or got his
patients to do so. Uncle Wolfi himself ate sparingly, I knew,
but not at all offensively.

Yet I could not see his advocating the equivalent of such fare
as hypocritical, for I knew Uncle to be sincere.

I also knew how little I understood of the science behind all
that Uncle had told me.

Still, give up at this point I could not, and go on with my
strange journey I must.

11 THE OLD WAY

I had enjoyed my reading. Yet, try as I might, I could not square that old way of eating with what was recommended today. Nowadays, any quantity of meat, especially red meat, was frowned on and any amount of fat in our food was a no-no. Babies should be given full-fat milk and even two-year-olds could enjoy, say, butter.

Then, for some reason that I couldn't fathom, the needs of young children were thought to change and, by five years old, they were being warned off butter at school. From toddlerhood onwards and for the rest of our lives, the advice was to partake of little meat – eating it three times a day was to court disaster – and to have less and less animal fat.

On the other hand, there was my remarkable Uncle Wolfi, who said 'nonsense' to all this and who made no secret about enjoying his meat. Leaving the fat on made it tasty, he said, and he was known to complain if the fat had been already cut off when the meat was bought. For Uncle maintained that, without enough fat, all would not be well either with our health or with our cooking!

Uncle said that as long as we stuck to traditional fats, fat in itself was not at all harmful and that too little fat could lead to a shortage of certain vitamins that were essential to us.

He said, too, that fat only became harmful if we overate in general, and especially if we overindulged in carbohydrate, a term covering starches and sugars generally. It was all very confusing.

What was I, a mere schoolgirl, to make of it all?

Uncle Wolfi had written a book about his life and work as a doctor, which had seen many editions. The book was called Leben ohne Brot, meaning 'life without bread', though Uncle didn't really mean no bread at all, not for everyone at least.

By 'bread', he was referring to the sugars and starches that occurred in the food we ate. And this included cereals! And he didn't mean life without any sugars and starches either, but life with only few.

Once, when I objected to his imprecise title, he just muttered something about poetic license. I have since wondered if this title was a piece of Uncle Wolfi's ironic humour and that he was trying to shock people into interest by using what for many of us was such an unthinkable proposition!

Uncle had kindly given me a copy of the first edition of his book. It was a very special present and I treasure it still.

In those days, my everyday German wasn't bad and I could speak it fairly well, but quite a lot of the German medical terms in this book were quite beyond me as yet.

However, I was able to decipher most of the introductory chapter and was pleased to see that it had photos of Vilhjalmur Stefansson and of a Copper Eskimo still living on the ancient diet, also a drawing of one of our ape-like predecessors.

It all felt very familiar and, now that I had read Stef's account of his visits to the Inuit, I was able to picture in my mind a genuine 'life without bread'.

It wasn't long before I was on the phone to Uncle Wolfi.

"Na, und? What now, little Sparrow?" was his greeting. That sounds unkind but I knew him well enough to see the familiar raised eyebrow and teasing smile that played around his lips when he answered my calls.

"In your book, Uncle, you say that the Inuit diet provided all the elements our ancestors needed for good healthy bodies. What did you mean exactly?"

"Think about it, Sparrow. Because the ancient peoples ate mostly animal food, this meant their diet consisted of mainly protein, some fat and a tiny bit of carbohydrate."

"So?"

"That, in my long considered opinion, is an ideal diet for Homo sapiens – ideal, mind you: I do not say sustainable nowadays or suited to the modern world."

"I don't think I'm much the wiser," I replied.

"Oh Sparrow, what on earth do you think our bodies are made of?" rejoined Uncle Wolfi. "Talk later, must go!"

Uncle seemed to be suggesting a connection between what our ancestors ate and what their bodies were made of, and this sparked me off on a new line of enquiry.

In biology lessons, I had learnt that all living things were made of a basic substance that contained protein, fat and carbohydrate and this now began to have meaning.

All living things must mean that it wasn't just animals, but also that all plants contained protein, fat and carbohydrate.

Well, I knew lamb chops had protein and fat in them – you could almost taste that they did – and that nuts and seeds did, too. But who would have thought there was fat in grass!

Moreover, I had seen a dog eating grass and then being sick and I had the feeling the same would happen to me. If so, grass wasn't much use to me for lunch, however much carbohydrate, fat or protein it contained!

It was different for a sheep or a cow with their special digestive arrangements, I thought.

Never forget you are a human and not a sheep, might have been Uncle Wolfi's words when I was playing that ape game so long ago.

I now began to grasp why Uncle had said we should leave grass to the grazers and eat the grazers instead!

But that wasn't the point. The point was to find out 'what on earth our bodies were made of', to use Uncle's words.

I am made of muscle, blood and bone and so on. Correction: I am made of what I eat, I mused, or rather from what I eat!

Logically, of course it had to be so – the things I ate were the only raw materials to hand.

I looked at my hands and wondered how my fingernails could possibly be made from cornflakes. I shook my head in bewilderment.

Stick to basics, Sparrow, I said to myself. Stick to protein, carbohydrate and fat!

Well, if the schoolbooks were correct, every living thing contained protein, carbohydrate and fat. Then I, as a living thing, had to contain protein, carbohydrate and fat, though in what proportions I did not know.

What is more, I ate living things – at least, I ate things that had once been living, whether a hamburger, a carrot or a baked potato. My food therefore also contained protein, carbohydrate and fat in varying proportions.

But what was I myself really made of?

In Mum's bookshelf, I found some biology books that had belonged to my grandmother. It surprised me that our own bodies consisted predominantly of water! Apparently nearly three-quarters of us was liquid and there was water in our cells and water between our cells.

As I felt so solid, I failed to imagine how I could be made mostly of water: it seemed so improbable.

Apart from water, it seemed that our bodies were also made of minerals and of very small amounts of the vitamins we are always hearing about, plus even less of the trace elements.

Otherwise, it seemed that our bodies consisted mainly of protein, some fat and a tiny bit of carbohydrate.

'Mainly of protein, some fat and a tiny bit of carbohydrate?' Oh dear, this did seem remarkably like how Uncle Wolfi had described the composition of the diet of our ancestral relatives.

Uncanny to say the least! Scary!

That evening, I got a quick word with Uncle Wolfi, who continued as though there had been no interruption in our earlier conversation.

"As I was saying, everything that we required to build and to power our bodies was present in our ancient diet.

Naturally, the ingredients of, say, wild boar still needed transposing into the ingredients that formed human beings as a unique species, that is into our own sort of protein, fat and carbohydrate.

Changing food into energy and body tissue involves a lot of complex chemical changes.

Nevertheless, I can't help feeling that, in those days, this conversion was relatively unproblematic."

And that was it! End of explanation!

So now to this business of changing protein, fat and carbohydrate into body tissue. I knew from Uncle about the need for protein to build and repair our bodies, but what did we want fat for?

I had been told often enough that fat is just what we don't want. Fat collects on our tummies and our thighs and we try our very best to get rid of it.

Just by looking round my classroom, I could see that fat collects in other places, too.

Yet in the old book that I was reading, fat was referred to as a normal, natural, even vital part of us.

It seemed our very brains were made mainly of fat – imagine having a brain made of fat and still being able to think!

The book said that fat was also the material from which our nerves were made. It seemed, too, that fat protected our organs from rubbing against or banging into each other.

Moreover, fat insulated us from the cold. Not only that, but fat was needed both for the forming of our trillions of little cells and for the work they did. Fat was even needed to build the body's messenger systems.

Therefore, from what I was reading, fat was vital to us and absolutely essential to our bodily construction.

We couldn't do without it; we couldn't live without it.

'Less fat', 'low fat', even 'no fat' claimed the television ads incessantly. Apparently, according to the ads, even some of this vital fat inside of us was a no-no and was to be got rid of as far as possible.

If this supposedly vital fat was deemed undesirable, well something had to be wrong. This was indeed bad.

If our brains turned out actually to be made, not just of any old fat, but of this very no-no fat, that was even worse!

I started worrying about what would happen if we got rid of too much fat from our bodies. For instance, if we ate too often foods specifically designed to 'lower the level' of those particular fats of which our cell walls are partly made, then what would happen to our cell walls?

And how would our poor brains be affected? Sparrow, just don't ask. It doesn't bear thinking about!

I was chuntering on to myself in this vein, when Mum came in. Overhearing me, she echoed:

"Sparrow, just don't ask," laughing at how I was talking to myself. "Stop worrying and leave all that to people like your Uncle Wolfi!

For all we know, the body can make its own special fats to keep things right. Let us hope so!

Personally, I don't buy that medicated margarine they advertise. I wouldn't have the stuff in the house! Now that I am starting to eat butter again, well, who ever heard of vegetable oils being popular in the Ice Age?"

"Anyone would think it was you and not Uncle who had written about life without bread," I commented dryly.

"In the meantime", said Mum ignoring my interruption, "your task is to try and understand for yourself something of what your Uncle is saying to you . . . well, and to the rest of us.

He is a clever fellow, you know, and didn't earn his distinction in medical science for nothing."

Good old Mum!

So I did my best to stop worrying and instead concentrated on learning about how the body changed the food we eat into energy.

12   A QUESTION OF FUEL

My mind went back to that wonderful time I had spent on the lake with Uncle Wolfi so many years ago.

He had made it clear that there were two good reasons for us eating food. These were firstly to keep ourselves in good repair and secondly to provide us with the necessary fuel for our existence.

I remember Uncle saying something about it mattering what kind of fuel our trillions of little cell engines used. He had talked of a primary fuel, which was particularly good at making energy and how, with the other two fuels, the little engines had to work twice as hard for the same output.

I knew by now that protein, carbohydrate and fat could all be used to make fuel. But which was the primary fuel for our bodies to use? My books at school weren't very clear about this, talking mostly of energy and calories.

In fact, I got the impression that sugar was thought to be our main fuel, especially for muscles. Certainly, I had often heard about filling up with carbohydrate before a race or taking Kendal mint-cake up mountains!

Then I thought of how the Masai could jogtrot all day in the heat of the African desert without carrying special top-up drinks or chocolate bars. The Masai were supposed to live on meat, blood and milk. I had seen photos of them and I thought they looked impressively strong and healthy.

I thought, too, of how Stef and his friend carried on life as normal for a whole year eating just the lean and fat of meat.

Neither Stef nor the Masai had much carbohydrate in their food, except the small amount that was in animal food.

Indeed, in ancient times, it seemed that for many people their energy was supplied entirely by animal food; for others this source was occasionally supplemented by plant food.

I felt confusion coming on me again. The Copper Eskimo in the Arctic did not eat cereals for breakfast. Not only that but they actually chose to go without breakfast on the day of a big hunt so that they had more energy for the hunt!

No breakfast meant more energy? To me, that didn't make any sense. Then there were the Inuit who carried on hunting for caribou or seals, even though they had not eaten for days.

This was so different from the way I conceived things to operate. I knew we ate to provide us with the fuel needed for us to make into energy, but I genuinely thought that everyone ate in order to give them the energy for the next few hours.

Well, less in my case. But, if I flopped in the meantime, I simply ate a few biscuits and I could then carry on with my homework, no probs.

It was obviously not like this for people living in the old way and who carried on hunting regardless.

Yet I – and most of my friends, for that matter – could scarcely get through morning school without feeling tired or hungry or both.

School catered for this by allowing us to bring in snacks.

Mum said that, when Granny was a girl, every day they all had a third of a pint of milk in the dining hall mid-morning and, if they had the required pennies, could buy an iced bun or a doughnut to go with it. Then it was only two hours to go until they were given a hot lunch of meat and veg, fish or cheese and potato pie, with a substantial pudding to come after. She said Granny also used to buy sweets to suck on the way home.

It was true that people who lived in the ancient way couldn't snack on popcorn or sweeties, because there weren't any. But what amazed me was that they didn't seem to need to do so.

Again something did not add up. And how could we have a constant supply of energy without constant eating?

It was OK for us because we had store cupboards and fridges and, for in-between times, we carried snacks in our school bags and most of my school friends kept sweets in their pockets.

But surely a nomadic people could neither store much food nor carry much food with them – or could they?

Here the magic word 'storage' went to work in my head. Could it be that our forbears actually carried their own supplies with them so that food was there whenever it was needed?

If so, did it mean that it was fat – their own body fat – that they mainly used for fuel?

Of course, it could be protein, but I had seen pictures of plump-faced Inuit people and – shush! – I remembered having read how the Kalahari bushmen grew big bottoms to carry their food stores in. These were also peoples who, in the twentieth century, were still living in a traditional manner.

Why wasn't it like that with us? Why were we so tied to mealtimes and snacks, I wondered?

In my class, there were girls with big bottoms who got just as hungry as I did. I knew of large adults, who must have had lots of stored fat, yet who didn't seem to be able to draw on it when they needed pepping up; in fact, they said they found it almost impossible to get the fat to budge at all.

The papers were full of slimming diets and how bad it was to be obese. Yet these 'primitive' peoples, given real luck with the hunt, ate until they were fit to bust. It didn't seem to do them any harm, so why did it hurt us?

I picked up the telephone: "Oh Uncle, why, why, oh why?" I almost groaned.

"You again, Sparrow? What can I do for you? I've only a couple of minutes."

"Oh Uncle, why was it good for the bushmen to obviously carry fat on their behinds and not us?

Why could the Copper Eskimo have a great feast of seal or whale meat, store fat but not get fat and not get in trouble with their health?

Why is it different for us?"

"Perhaps," said Uncle Wolfi slowly, "life was a little different then?"

"Yes, yes, I know that there was a long period of time in which you needed to be healthy enough just to survive: a time when there were no hospitals or drugs, a time before bread, baked beans or potato crisps," I said impatiently.

There was a distinct pause at the other end of the telephone but I grumbled on:

"Personally, I don't think nature foresaw the 21st century!"

"Perhaps, it was the coming of agriculture that nature did not foresee!" rejoined Uncle Wolfi, laughing. "Or, just perhaps, it is not nature's job to foresee but rather to adapt and evolve?"

"Yes, but . . ." I began.

"One moment, Sparrow! Have you considered the fact that the bodies of your primitive people could still be working as nature intended?

Remember that the long period of time you speak of lasted over 100,000 years. It is a real possibility that the system on which the bodies of early Homo sapiens operated – of our own kin, that is – was in place for at least that long."

"And still is?" I asked tentatively, overawed at this thought. Fleeting memories of those special Austrian holidays of years ago passed across my mind.

"Chickens?" I suggested in a half-whisper.

"Genuine biological adaptation can be a very slow business, you know.

So why don't you forget today and keep learning about the ground plan, as it were, that is how our bodies still appear to work according to the needs of times gone by.

I think you'll find it most interesting. Do excuse me: I must go, Sparrow. Duty calls!" so saying, Uncle rang off.

Forget today, Uncle Wolfi had said, and learn about how our bodies used to work in those far off pre-cereal times all those thousands of years ago. So it was back to the old times, back to times of scarcity, irregularity of food supply, of sudden plenty or near famine.

More especially, I was to find out how we functioned on the diet of protein, some fat and a tiny amount of carbohydrate, which Uncle had said was the normal diet of human beings in those days of long ago.

Was this another of Uncle's mysterious puzzles? If so, this one was a real challenge.

Liking puzzles, I eagerly returned to Granny's old books to see if I could find some answers to the question of fuel.

Yes, energy was necessary for heating our bodies and also all other bodily activities like running, eating, going to the loo, digestion and playing football – or maybe hunting buffalo?

As a fuel to provide this energy, nature would surely use the most efficient fuel. I had already decided this couldn't be carbohydrate, since there wasn't enough of it around.

It wasn't long before I found confirmation that our primary fuel was indeed fat. Not only was fat more effective but was just over twice as efficient as carbohydrate or protein.

Moreover, our little engines loved it best and, believe it or not, our body's muscles – and this included our hearts – preferred to run mostly on the energy from fat. Yes, it really said that fat was the best fuel for our hearts!

Talking of hearts, in my own heart of hearts I was hoping to prove Uncle Wolfi mistaken in this matter, but it looked like I was on a loser.

What is more, with fat as its main fuel, the body operated happily and competently with a steady stream of energy independent of the last meal. Yes, a 'steady stream of energy independent of the last meal' was written in black and white.

And had not Uncle Wolfi said as much years ago?

This meant that the insides of our Ice-Age brethren were truly organised in a marvellous way that ensured there was no premature flag if food was not immediately to hand.

How clever! Come to think of it, it had to be so, or how could people's hearts keep ticking steadily throughout the night? I felt abashed not to have thought of that before.

I read on with enthusiasm. At a time when fat necessarily provided most of our fuel needs, nature in her wisdom had indeed made it possible for our forbears to carry their own fuel supplies with them as body fat. This was just as I had guessed.

Moreover, fat inside the body was easily stored and just as

91

easily accessed when needed for energy. In those days, fat was popped in and out of storage in the twinkling of an eye, with our little cell engines chugging away in microseconds.

I learnt that, in the main, fat from the food was taken up for use by the cells more quickly and by a different process than that of either protein or carbohydrate. I say 'in the main', as a little sweetness could be taken up directly from the mouth, but then how much sweetness was there in the ancient diet?

I could see that, for a people who needed to obtain their energy predominantly from fat, this ability to absorb fat fairly quickly made sense, especially as there couldn't always have been a great deal of fat in their diet in the first place.

And aren't a lot of wild animals rather lean in springtime? A walrus would be fine, but a March hare? I could see why, though I personally would not relish such fare, fatty foods like brain and bone marrow used to be much prized.

So yes, in ancient times, fat would have been the primary fuel. However, the body also used protein and carbohydrate for fuel. Protein would have been no problem as there would have been plenty in the food, but whence came the carbohydrate?

Eating meat – or eating animal food generally – would have supplied plenty of protein and some fat.

However, just as there was only a tiny bit of carbohydrate in our own make-up, so there was only a tiny bit of carbohydrate in animal food.

I had read that this was present as a type of starch. Yet apparently the bloodstream needed sugar.

This conundrum interested me.

"Hey, Mum!" I shouted.
"I can't hear you, I am in the kitchen!" called back Mum.

I was so excited that I actually got out of my chair and went to find her.

"Guess what I've found out!" I said proudly.

"Well?" said Mum.

"It's something that they usually don't admit," I exclaimed. "Do you know what starch is?" I quizzed but didn't wait for a reply. "Starch is just a lot of sugar molecules lumped together! Isn't that wonderful?"

"Starch is just a lot of sugar molecules lumped together?" repeated Mum. "So all the body has to do is to break the starch down again and it becomes sugar?"

"You must admit, Mum, that it's cool!"

"Yet on the radio they are saying that now sugar is bad for us, starchy food is to form the basis of our diet!"

"Yes, Mum, it is a con! A real con! But don't worry, Mum, the ancient people based their diet mostly on protein and fat."

"I was thinking of today," replied Mum.

"Today comes later!" I said reassuringly.

Mum just looked at me:

"And you, my child, as you won't have touched the sugar bowl, can pig on pasta and still feel virtuous. Clever!"

Perhaps I should have kept my findings to myself!

"Has this discovery a particular relevance, I wonder?" asked Mum, while she stirred the goulash.

"Ah yes!" I said, quickly reverting to what I had been studying. "For a start, it means that the ancient people could make sugar for their bloodstream from the small amounts of animal starch in their dinner.

You know, Mum, how sugar is needed for brains and so on. Well, our forebears needed enough blood sugar for the everyday running of their bodies – not a lot, but enough; so some came from breaking down this starch and the rest could be manufactured by converting to sugar some of the protein present in their diet, as well as the protein left over from body waste such as dead cells etc."

"You mean a sort of cleaning up device. I call it useful recycling," commented Mum.

I wanted to tell Mum that there were other complicated mechanisms that could be activated to help, say the brain if it lacked sugar, but I hadn't really understood them myself.

In any case, she had gone off to the garden to pick chard.

How beautifully thought-through it all was!

You see, the body had no means of storing sugar as such. For emergencies, though, the body did keep a small amount of this starch, which was stored in the liver and in the muscles and which could be broken down to provide blood sugar when it was really necessary.

This was one of the built-in mechanisms for times of danger, for example to give an extra burst of energy for that fast sprint away from a rhino or polar bear. In such a case, the muscles needed to use sugar rather than fat.

I particularly noted that this storage of starch for use as sugar was not designed for everyday use. Rather it was one of the body's reserves – an emergency resource only to be called on in cases of real stress. This felt important.

The storage of starch was also a valuable failsafe measure for when food was in short supply.

In times of starvation, when no food at all was available, these stores of starch got quickly used up. The body then had no alternative but to fall back on using not just its own deep body fat but also its own essential body protein to cover its needs for energy, including its need for blood sugar.

This was why people who were starving became so thin and weak: the body used its own actual tissues to create the energy even just to stay alive. Grim!

All in all, the bodies of our immediate forbears really did seem to be organised with the expectation of little carbohydrate being present in food.

It fitted, too, that there was a built-in arrangement to restrict the amount of sugar to be carried in the bloodstream. Not so with fat: in order to transport fat round the body, there was a lot of latitude as to the amount of fat which the bloodstream could carry safely at any one time. There was even a little reservoir to help digest extra fat, if needed.

This suited both the type and the variable quantity of food our forbears could expect.

It meant their system was geared to cope with their usual moderate or sparse intake, such as a meagre ration of one ptarmigan per family or not even that.

Yet it was also geared to cope with the occasional big influx of fat and protein, such as a feast of wild ox, in which case they tanked up with all they could eat, to first satiate their appetites and then to save against a rainy day.

Struggling through Uncle's first edition, I could see that there were all sorts of controls to oversee the smooth working of the internal goings-on, with many messengers to ensure proper communication between the various parts of the body, all sorts of adjustments here and there as needed.

And there was a difficult bit about a balance; something about an equilibrium to be kept between the use of substance to produce energy and the use of energy to build substance.

It seemed that a suitable diet promoted co-operation between our various body systems and so ensured that this important balance prevailed harmoniously.

In short, what I had grasped from all my reading so far was that the body was kind and wonderfully built to be healthy and, come what may, to make the best of things.

"It seems that on our ancient diet, the workings of the body would have run smoothly. What is different these days in the way our bodies are supposed to work?" I asked Uncle later.

"Perhaps there is no fundamental difference," he said.

"But I thought you said nature's job was to move from what went before into what suited the new surroundings at the time?" I commented hopefully.

"In my own opinion, Sparrow, there has not been enough time for our bodies to adapt sufficiently to the very changed conditions of today."

"Now you tell me!" I said a little testily.

"But think of all you have just learnt!" said Uncle with his usual good humour.

"Well, you said to study the old way and, as far as I can make it out from what Granny's old books say, it seems that our bodies would work really well and harmoniously on our ancient diet of protein, some fat and a tiny bit of carbohydrate."

"I agree with you, but as to a harmonious balance prevailing, I feel there is one important proviso – that the diet doesn't exceed a certain level of carbohydrate."

"And if it does, Uncle Wolfi, what then?"

13 HOPE

It was about this time that Uncle Wolfi paid one of his rare visits up North. Mother was out when he turned up on our doorstep with a big bunch of flowers in his arms.

"For Sparrow," he said, handing me the flowers with a slight bow, "for my budding little scholar!" I couldn't tell if he was joking, but then I never could.

Here he was: the same Uncle Wolfi, still upright, slim and immaculately dressed, almost dapper, the same droll smile that I remembered so well.

I asked Uncle in and, taking his coat, offered him an armchair by the fire. It was wintertime and he stretched out his long legs gratefully.

"Coal?" he queried. I nodded and took a seat nearby.

"Perhaps I should call you Wolfgang, now that I'm getting older," I ventured. "I'm fifteen now."

"Please don't: it would make me feel old, too! And then I might start calling you my old pigeon!" I let that pass.

"So Uncle Wolfi it is, then. Well, I think that your idea that the food we eat should be suited to our inner workings is remarkably sensible."

I had been thinking about this for hours before his visit:

"As you know, I have been reading up about evolution and also about the design of our bodies."

"I'm going to enjoy this," he said softly.

"But what happens when we have 'too much of a good thing', as you put it? And recently you mentioned balance and an important proviso, what did you mean?"

"Ah!" exclaimed Uncle. "Perhaps you would first offer your remarkably sensible Uncle a cup of tea after all his travelling?"

"I'm sorry, Uncle, yes of course, it's just that . . ." I was saying as I disappeared into the kitchen.

When I came back, Uncle Wolfi smiled. "Thank you. Most welcome. And how's Mutti?" he asked, as I poured the tea.

'Mutti' was what we both called Mum when I was in Austria.

"Mum's fine," I said, adding confidentially, "guess what! I noticed that she had been peering into the book you gave me – the lovely old one with the picture of the ape-man – and soon afterwards I found that there was full-cream milk in the fridge.

I didn't say anything, but a little later I heard her telling a neighbour how, on advice from a hospital for something or other, she had been 'low fat' for 17 years. She said she had never had digestive troubles before that time, but on and off ever since, oh dear . . .!

I pricked up my ears to hear her say that, now that she's cut down on bread a little and put butter back on the table, her insides are a lot better."

"It figures," said Uncle, nodding slowly.

"And she finished by saying 'the old boy certainly has something!'"

I glanced at Uncle to see if he was offended, but his eyes were twinkling just as they used to.

Anyway, old boy seemed somehow right because, although he really was quite old, there was still something boyish about the way he used to tease people and enjoy little jokes.

In one of his many letters, he had told me how he sometimes

liked to provoke his illustrious colleagues with some new theory of his.

"And I gave up sugar in my tea for Lent!" I added proudly.

"Good lass, that's a start," he said approvingly and declining with a small gesture of his hand the plate of custard creams I was offering.

When he had finished his cup of tea, he looked at me with an enquiring smile.

"Where shall we start?"

"I've heard about sugar causing problems with our health, but what I really want to know, Uncle, is why cereals cause trouble," I said, eager to get going. "And also what trouble they cause."

"Ah!" he said again. "In my opinion, it is not just cereal, but an overload of carbohydrate from any source.

It is interesting, though, isn't it that archaeologists can tell whether old skeletons date to the Ice Age or more recently by the condition of their teeth? It seems that when cereal entered our diet, so did tooth decay!"

"You mean it's not just sugary food that rots our teeth?" I exclaimed surprised.

"Oh, both cereals and tooth decay entered our lives long before sugar did!" affirmed Uncle Wolfi.

Uncle considered for a moment then added: "Of course, generally speaking, it is difficult to know exactly which bit of our bodies is upset by which items of food. Not only that but, in our modern life, there are so many factors other than food involved that it is difficult to tease causes apart. For example, pollution, stress, lack of exercise and so on may worsen a particular disease."

"I can see that," I said.

"I could not change modern life. Nor could I feed my patients even more of the suspected foodstuffs to see if they got increased trouble! That would be unethical as well as unfair. So how was I to prove or even demonstrate that the cause of such and such an ailment was eating too much carbohydrate – whether bread or sugar?

In the end, I decided that one way of identifying a root cause might be to leave everything else the same and merely reduce the overload of sugars and starches to see what happened. That is the approach I took.

Or was it a biology lesson you were looking for?" he asked, adjusting his legs a little.

"Both," I said hopefully.

When Uncle Wolfi spoke in English, which he did well, he spoke slowly and carefully. Unfortunately, I cannot replicate his lovely Austrian accent on paper which, for me, was very much part of him.

It was good to be with him again and when Uncle now began to get restless, said he had been sitting for hours in the train and didn't I think it was time for his half hour's walk, it felt just like old times. So we got our coats on and walked together down to the beach.

"You call this a beach?" he asked, gazing at the long expanse of salt marsh and the distant sea. "I see you have a cave!"

It was a sizeable cave in the low limestone cliff that rose near to where we were standing. I had often played there in the past with friends. It was fun shouting into it to hear the echoes.

"That cave of yours takes me back to a turning point in my thinking. It was half a lifetime ago," he said, smiling at the recollection, "and I had driven to the South of France to try out my new sports car."

I could see Uncle Wolfi owning such a fast car when he was younger.

"Seeing the prehistoric cave paintings at Lascaux and Trois Frères – amazingly vibrant paintings of game animals such as deer, wild horses and aurochs – is what woke me to the reality of our ancient diet and its dependence on animals.

Yet we consign our magnificent ancestors to prehistory! Don't you think it odd that history only starts when cereals entered the picture?"

What an idea! I was all ears.

"As you know, at the time I was not in the best of health!" he continued.

"I don't think you were, Uncle," I said, responding to his understatement.

I knew for a fact that he had been quite a wreck: had dicky hips, splitting headaches, bad teeth and a narky temper and could scarcely do his work any longer.

Yet here he was still working in his old age!

"But do tell me more about when you tried your own diet on yourself and went cereal-free for four years."

"It was soon after going to the caves. I had been a lover of good rich fare – and you know yourself what lovely pastries we make in Austria.

One day, I cut right down on such delicacies, also on all cereals, as you know. I noticed with interest that my headaches gradually subsided, my digestion improved as did my dental health, I was much calmer and I no longer caught colds easily.

101

What is more, the trouble I used to have in my hip joints vanished like magic."

"I thought you didn't believe in magic, Uncle."

"Sparrow, you are getting too much for an old man!"

"To please you, let me be more accurate", said Uncle Wolfi after a pause. "Over the following few months, it was the pain and stiffness in my hips that just melted away and that, as you can imagine, felt like magic!

The actual bony changes are still there even today yet, once I was well established on the diet, they no longer stopped me doing a little skiing or playing tennis.

I even started looking the sportsman but this, I'm fairly sure, came more from the diet than from my moderate level of physical activity."

I looked at Uncle Wolfi admiringly. He was a tryer!

"The diet gave me many years of freedom, maybe twenty, maybe more, but eventually I did need one hip doing," he confessed. "Perhaps I brought it on myself by playing too much tennis? And these days, my other hip does occasionally remind me of its old trouble.

But we don't want to talk about me, do we? Let's walk on a little to get a better view of the sea."

We walked for a while over the springy grass, carefully weaving our way around the dips and pools. It was a lovely day; the sun was already low and the colours in the late afternoon sky were glorious.

"So, Uncle Wolfi, to get really well, you think we should eat mainly meat like our prehistoric relatives?"

"Did I say so?" asked Uncle with some surprise.

"No, well, not exactly – and, in the past, I have seen you eat ice cream and even pudding!"

"Quite. You see, my tastes are modern! Wouldn't you say so, Sparrow?" he said with a somewhat challenging smile.

But I was not going let his joking distract me.

"Then, Uncle, your basic message is simply: go easy on the carbohydrates," I declaimed, jumping over a pool.

"Nothing is quite that simple, Sparrow," said Uncle Wolfi with mild reproof.

"But it is agreed we need protein and I know that you don't disapprove of people eating fat, especially traditional fats, do you Uncle? That is, as long as they keep their carbohydrate intake reasonable."

"True," he acknowledged, and we walked on.

I was the first to break the silence.

"I have been wondering about this business of reasonable. But what is a reasonable intake of carbohydrate, Uncle Wolfi?" I asked, full of curiosity.

"A fair question. Reasonable? Reasonable for whom and under what circumstances? Or do you mean ideal?

Let me tell you what I find ideal for therapeutic purposes and that is something like the level of carbohydrate in our ancient diet but a little more."

"It can't have been much!" I exclaimed with some apprehension.

"This level of carbohydrate might have seemed a severe restriction to some people," admitted Uncle Wolfi, "but what you have to realise is that, as a doctor, I was dealing with patients, many of whom were seriously ill.

By the time people came to me, as a Consultant in Internal

Medicine, they were very often already considerably damaged by carbohydrate overload.

It was no easy job to treat people so damaged and to get them well again. I found that I needed to use such strict measures to get results.

Perhaps my therapeutic level kick-started the healing process and promoted a change to a more appropriate gear?"

Uncle seemed to like analogies with engines and cars.

"It is interesting, however, that for others who weren't so ill to start with, even a slight reduction in carbohydrate could start turning them around," continued Uncle Wolfi after a pause.

"I noticed you weren't surprised that Mum was feeling better," I commented, "even though she only cut down a little."

"A case in point," he replied. "You see, it is the digestive tract that is in direct contact with food and so, if carbohydrates have offended, it is often the first part of the body to make its protest felt.

Fortunately, if the case is not too serious, it is also the first to be pacified when the situation is reversed and carbohydrates are reduced.

Importantly, I have found that adding fat not only satiates but also calms the digestive tract. I used to pronounce quite boldly that there was no healing of the gut without fat."

"Guts need fat!" I echoed.

"Such a statement used to get me into such trouble with my colleagues, but I still think there is a lot of truth in it."

We walked and talked and had become so engrossed that we did not notice time passing until I shivered a little.

"Come on, the sun is almost down and it's getting colder.

Let's go back!" said Uncle Wolfi.

As we returned along the lane, Uncle Wolfi told me about the good things that happened when people went on his diet.

Apparently, there was not just improvement in their medical condition, but many of his patients found benefits seemingly unrelated to their known complaint.

People reported sleeping better and, amongst other things, catching fewer infections; having less need for the dentist and having warmer hands and feet.

As he mentioned warm hands, Uncle Wolfi glanced at me enquiringly.

"I know, I know," I sighed. "Yes, they are still cold, but that is just the way I am."

"Na, ja," was Uncle's only comment.

"But that wasn't all," Uncle Wolfi continued, "many patients found they suffered from less bloating of their abdomens; their stomachs were happier, as you can imagine.

People found that their skin was in better condition and, moreover, that their corns disappeared!"

"That's amazing!" I exclaimed.

"And it wasn't just corns. A better mental disposition was experienced and patients tended to feel better in themselves generally. I have verified all this during consultations.

Last but not least, most people found that they needed to eat less often and also ate less in quantity than they previously did, which, though welcome, quite surprised them

Patients gained hope from these various benefits and I'm sure this encouraged them to persevere with the diet," he concluded.

"To me, Uncle Wolfi, these blessings seem very similar to many that you experienced in your own life," I observed. "I am impressed."

At suppertime, we had local roast beef and Uncle found it very good and ate heartily, but he graciously declined the Yorkshire pudding, the roast and boiled potatoes and the fried Brussels sprouts with ginger and garlic.

Uncle Wolfi looked at the roast parsnips doubtfully.

"Are they vegetables?" he asked.

Mum assured him that they were.

It turned out he had never seen a parsnip before, so I went and looked up parsnip in my German dictionary and got a word equivalent to a country bumpkin! How we laughed!

Uncle did accept a small portion of trifle for dessert.

Our serious conversation, though, was over for the day and I had to await the morning for our next instalment.

14 THE NEW NORM?

Next morning, Uncle looked well rested. Mum enquired what he would like for breakfast.

"Coffee would be fine, thank you. You see, I am not accustomed to eat much during the day, but I do enjoy a good evening meal."

"Are you sure you won't accept anything else, Wolfgang?" asked Mum, feeling a bit inadequate as a hostess.

"I would accept a cup of cream to go with my black coffee. That would be very nice."

In the event, Uncle Wolfi also ate a boiled egg with butter and we felt that at least he had something in his tummy for his long return trip to London via Cambridge, where he was to meet a colleague to discuss a research proposal.

"So what questions have you for me before I leave, little Miss Why-Why?" he said, turning to me once he had finished.

"Carbohydrates again, please," I said without hesitation.

"Now, you have been learning about the Ice Age and I see that you have got the message very clearly that, in those days, there was little carbohydrate in our diet . . .?"

"Yes, and what I can't understand is, well, why everybody doesn't know your 'secret' about diet needing to suit the design of our bodies – it is so obvious!"

Then I heard in my mind the distant barbaric yawp of the spotted hawk: that's one reason, I thought.

I pictured the shelves and shelves of starchy and sweet food in our local shop and the temptations in the window of the local bakery, and thought of the more-ish nature of sweets, cakes, toast, breakfast cereal and pasta: there's another reason.

"From the expression on your face, you are beginning to answer your own question!" said Uncle, who had been watching me intently.

"There is something I can't make out, Uncle Wolfi. It's about where we actually get our energy from. On the ancient diet, it was fat, and the fat came both from the food people ate and from stores in their bodies.

Nowadays, if the operation of our bodies has stayed the same, it should still be fat, shouldn't it? According to both you and the old biology books, it is the principal and most efficient energy provider.

Yet, according to our school textbooks, even though little carbohydrate can be stored in our body, it is sugar and not fat which is supposed to be our main source of energy, at least for our muscles.

Do you think that is why we are told to make carbohydrates the basis of our diet? And if there has been no big change in the way our bodies work since those days – and you said not – then what is going on?"

There was a lull in our conversation. Uncle was leaning back in his chair. He had long slender fingers and was now slowly tapping the fingertips of one hand against the fingertips of the other, as though he were thinking.

"You, Sparrow, have put your finger on a source of serious misunderstanding.

Over the years I have noticed a worrying tendency to reclassify according to what happens in everyday life and not according to our origins or our inherent design."

"So?" I said, not quite seeing this as an answer to my question.

"So," he replied, only Uncle pronounced it 'zoh'. "So . . ." he repeated. Here Uncle sighed:

"Willingness to eat something doesn't mean . . ."

"That dogs should eat too much chocolate!" I put in.

"Quite!" agreed Uncle, nodding.

Then Uncle Wolfi sat upright and alert: "Take the domestic cat, for example. There is no dispute that cats of all sizes are carnivorous by origin and design and still are so in the wild. Think tigers, lions and lynxes.

But now that the much-loved domestic cat is willing to eat appropriately flavoured cat biscuits, even some vets are designating cats as omnivores."

I grinned at this:

"Well, in a sense Uncle Wolfi, they are omnivores if, like us, they eat biscuits as well as meat!"

"Oh Sparrow, can't you see that such a practice takes no account at all of the costs of this so-called omnivory to the cat's health?

Such a way of eating is so foreign to the bodies of cats that they are becoming ever more subject to disease – and curiously enough to our own modern diseases. The thing is, sooner or later, this mixed diet makes the cats ill . . ."

"And the vets rich?" I asked, thinking of all the medicines my best friend's cat had to take.

"Precisely! And perhaps the same process is happening as regards our own main source of energy? What do you say?

Moreover, like with the domestic cat, it ignores the costs to our health?"

"I don't quite get your drift, Uncle," I said.

Then my thoughts went to my family and how ill my grandmother had been and with the very same disease as my friend's cat. The cost of omnivory? No, surely not!

"You can't mean you question humans being omnivorous, Uncle, surely?"

"It's the 'omni' bit which I question," growled Uncle Wolfi somewhat savagely.

"Omnis, all or every," I remarked, displaying my prowess at Latin.

"Your Latin is OK but how is your logic nowadays?" asked Uncle, still gruff.

"Not bad", I said modestly.

"Take this:

Because we actually do something, therefore it is normal.
Because it is normal, therefore it is natural.
Because it is natural, therefore we ought to do that thing.

Who steps back and questions the logic?"

I had no answer to that:

"I pass," I said.

"Yes, we may well be able to supplement our basic diet on occasion, or even on a regular basis, with food from the plant kingdom," continued Uncle, "Perhaps it is thought of as the new norm? But the classification 'omnivore' MUST NOT MISLEAD US INTO BELIEVING THAT WE HUMANS CAN EAT ANYTHING AND EVERYTHING WITH IMPUNITY, AND ESPECIALLY IN ANY QUANTITY.

I, myself, am sure that we cannot!"

This last speech was declaimed loud and decisively, after which Uncle fell silent again, ruminating about something.

15   THE BEST JOKE YET

"Perhaps it is time for a little biology?" I suggested gently.

"A good idea. That might help you understand a little more about sources of energy," said Uncle, brightening.

We were still sitting at the breakfast table and we now both got up and moved into the living room.

"Na, und? Well?" I said teasingly to pre-empt him.

"Na, und" repeated Uncle Wolfi and, changing language mid-sentence, he continued:

"I think we have established that the advent of cereals, a food item full of concentrated starch, introduced a gradually increasing amount of carbohydrate into our diet.

Lately, there has been a dramatic increase."

I was thoughtful: "But, Uncle, we do have the capacity to digest some starch."

"True, and both plant starch and animal starch."

"If we can digest it, why does the increase matter, Uncle?" I wondered.

"This is where the biology comes in. It matters because when we eat carbohydrate, it reaches our bloodstream as sugar, as you know."

"Yes, I was reading about starch being just a mass of sugar molecules."

"That's right, and so carbohydrate of virtually any sort, whether it starts out as sugar or starch on the plate, still enters our bloodstream as sugar: blood sugar, glucose.

You see, it's not just sugar that makes a difference to our blood sugar levels – that's what so many people fail to realise, including, I'm sorry to say, some of my own profession.

Yet this is of fundamental importance to us all, and especially to those with blood sugar problems."

"And?" I asked, encouraging him to continue.

"And eating cereal or any other food high in carbohydrate, say, eating a bowlful of porridge or sweet fruit, can create more sugar than our bloodstream was used to receiving on our ancient diet."

"Doughnuts?" I queried.

"Doughnuts, for instance," he confirmed, "even having three croissants for breakfast, not to mention very generous portions of Schokoladensoufflé after dinner", said Uncle Wolfi, looking at me knowingly.

He then stopped.

"Let me see," said Uncle slowly. "I know that you are already aware that the bloodstream can carry safely only a certain amount of sugar at any one time, so why don't you put your little enquiring mind to work. I'll ask you the questions!"

I quaked a little but kept silent.

"If your body had too much of something it didn't expect and didn't want, what would it do?" he asked.

"It would try to get rid of it, of course."

"Go on!"

"Well, I could be sick or," I suggested, thinking back to Stefansson's experience, "get the trots?"

"Yes, that would work to immediately empty your stomach or your bowels and you would be very aware of it! But if that something was in your bloodstream, which you cannot usually feel because it is right inside of you?"

It was my turn to say "Ah!" But then I thought of our kidneys: "I'd pee it out!"

"As an emergency reaction to such a surprise, that is exactly what a traditional Inuit would have done when encountering 'white man's food' for the first time.

Not expecting a rise in blood sugar, the 'guards' were asleep but, in this unusual situation, the kidneys, which are never off duty and which filter the bloodstream night and day, did the honours, as it were. Well done, Sparrow!"

"However," continued Uncle Wolfi: "too many encounters with extra sugar in the bloodstream and this would change. Ship's biscuits are not what the body would have wanted to receive but, say, the person has developed a taste for them and is now eating them every day?

Wouldn't a regular addition to the bloodstream, which was unwanted, require a rethink? In that case, what would your body now do with the sugar it didn't want there?"

I reflected for a moment:

"It would think 'I don't want all this horrid extra stuff. It is OK in the right amount but there is just too much of it, so maybe I could make use of it in some way: change it, store it, anything rather than have it in my bloodstream!'" and I mimicked the indignation my body would feel.

Uncle smiled:

"And this is precisely what it did – and still does. To rid the bloodstream of any surplus sugar, over safe limits that is, the body puts the extra either to immediate use or it makes it into storable commodities for future use."

"You see, you were quite right when you said that the body does its best for us in any particular situation.

Given our beginnings as a species, our original design was necessarily organised around the principle of conservation and recycling. Our body was therefore programmed to cherish every morsel of nourishment that we ate. Potential food would otherwise be going to waste."

"Yes, it would be," I agreed, feeling quite pleased with myself.

I thought that this was the end of the lesson, but no, there was a 'but'.

"But," Uncle was saying, "there are one or two slight snags to overcome: namely, in a body that has limited natural use for carbohydrate of any sort and, in any case, cannot store sugar as such, how is it to achieve either use or storage, I wonder?"

"I know," I said, scarcely refraining from putting my hand up as though I was at school. "It could burn the extra sugar as fuel!"

"It could – and it does – but to do so on a regular basis or in any quantity is not without problems of its own," replied Uncle Wolfi. "Once it becomes a main fuel . . ."

"More trouble?" I queried uneasily, for I had hoped that if excess sugar in the blood could be burnt safely as our main fuel, this would solve my fat versus sugar fuel dilemma.

"Don't worry about that now", said Uncle reassuringly, "just try to think it through. Any ideas as to where and in what form the body could store the excess?"

"I did read that the liver converts sugar in the blood to starch. I suppose it might be able to convert a little more and add it to its existing stores? If pushed, maybe the muscles could accommodate a little more of this starch, too?"

"Good so far! Yes, some of the extra sugar could be used as fuel straightaway and a little could be stored as starch in the muscles and liver, though not a lot, mind you.

There is a third possibility – and here is the rub – for the body also has the capacity to convert sugar into fat."

"You don't say, Uncle!" Now this was something!
I knew fat could be stored as fat because that was the old way with the Inuit and the bushmen, but I had missed this bit of the puzzle.
"But, niece, I do say," replied Uncle.
"You mean that the body can also change sugar in the blood into fat? No, don't answer: let me guess!"
I started jumping up and down in my seat with anticipation:
"The body then uses this fat as fuel, which, on the whole, is the fuel it prefers to use in any case? Dilemma solved!"
"Ah, yes and no!" said Uncle Wolfi not reciprocating my excitement. "You see, whether the fat can actually be used in that way depends . . . "
"Depends?"
"Well, it depends for a start on the modesty of the eater in respect of carbohydrate, and we'll come to that in due course.
Certainly it can store the fat it creates from sugar, and can do so if necessary in large quantities."

Uncle Wolfi was serious but I began to giggle. In fact, I was so amused that I didn't even hear what Uncle had just said.
"Oh Uncle, it cracked me up before to learn that, whereas our bodies don't welcome much sugar, there are even special arrangements to deal with the fat we eat, so that the 'nasty' fat gets into the bloodstream quickly enough! In fact, these special

arrangements are to please the fat-hungry cells who want it always on tap to give them the energy they need."

"I think the blood puts it into the fat tissue so that it is ready for immediate use," put in Uncle.

"And it seems the bloodstream can cope - and safely so - with quantities of fat, whether you are pigging on seal blubber or the back fat of reindeer. What feasting!" I said, pulling a face and remembering what I had read about Arctic life.

"Pigging on pork or bacon fat might be a more apt phrase, Sparrow," chuckled Uncle Wolfi. "As for feasting, we must never forget about the lean times and also about famine."

"You must admit that it is funny, though, Uncle! We are not supposed to eat too much sugar and are instructed to eat more carbohydrate instead. And what does the body do? It turns the carbohydrate into sugar anyway! It's quite wonderful!

Then there is all this fuss about not eating fat! But the body itself turns a lot of the sugar resulting from the carbohydrate into fat anyway. It's rich! So we may as well have eaten fat in the first place," I reasoned, still laughing.

"I only wish more people could see the joke", said Uncle, dryly and without a smile. "In fact, one wonders if any real consideration for health comes into their thinking."

"What's more," I continued" I thought it funny enough when I found out that, although it's supposed to be risky to eat much animal protein and positively dangerous to eat much animal fat, it is precisely animal protein and fat that we – that is our bodies – are actually composed of!"

"Well, if you were made of plant fat and plant protein, it wouldn't be you, would it! Welcome to the animal kingdom, my little soya bean!" said Uncle wryly.

116

"But that we can turn the carbohydrate we eat, not just into fat when it gets inside of us, but into animal fat at that, is the best joke yet." I said, bursting into uncontrollable laughter.

Uncle waited for me to calm down.

"I mean, I mean," I stuttered: "You couldn't make it up! All that hoo-ha about avoiding animal fat, so what do we do? We stuff ourselves full of sugar and starch only to end up full of animal fat anyway!"

"I'm glad you see the irony," said Uncle Wolfi, as I wiped the tears of merriment from my eyes.

16 TIPPING THE BALANCE

Uncle now stood up and walked round the room.

"Clever isn't it, rendering an unwanted substance such as extra blood sugar potentially useful!" he began.

"Very green," I readily acknowledged, trying to pay attention once again.

"In both senses of the word!" said Uncle with a teasing smile. "It recycles, yes, but the measure is naïve – or should I say it does not readily work to our advantage – as even the fatty tissue can be stretched!

That is a pun, you see," he added, seeing my puzzlement. "Well, the fat cells do in fact stretch to accommodate the extra fat to be stored and they also grow in number.

Moreover, neither the liver nor the muscles have any desire to store much extra starch. All this is fair enough if these measures are required only occasionally . . ." Uncle broke off mid-sentence to ask:

"Can you spot any possible problems, little Sparrow?"

I reflected for a moment: "Maybe, just like the bloodstream with all that extra sugar, the muscles would get irritated and think 'I don't want all this horrid extra stuff. It is OK in the right amount but there is just too much of it'?

I suppose the only answer would be to do lots of exercise and sport to force the muscles to use rather than store the unwanted extra starch?

I know that skinny rabbits like me can have too much zip! Mum often says 'for God's sake can't you ever sit still?'"

Uncle Wolfi smiled:

"Go on."

"And I have been wondering why very fat people aren't always bouncing with energy: they should be with all that stored fat at their disposal. I can't make it out."

"Can you guess?"

"I'm still trying to get my head round it," I said quite honestly and, as he was still pacing round the living room, I added:

"Uncle Wolfi, I am wondering whether you would like a proper walk? Do you have time?"

"I don't have to leave for an hour or so. Yes, let's go."

In no time, well wrapped up against the cold, Uncle Wolfi and I were off through the hazel copse at the end of our road and on towards the long ridge of mixed woodland.

Here, a pair of peregrine falcons roosted; I had seen father and son carry off white doves from the roof of our neighbour's house. I don't think I would have liked to be a real sparrow with those birds around!

Soon we reached the wood and were ambling together through paths deep with leaf mould. It smelt wonderful and Uncle looked happy.

"In those days, the guards were only called out when there was a real emergency!" he said, quite out of the blue.

"Sorry?" I said, not catching on.

We had arrived at a clearing from where there was a pleasing view over the bay and surrounding area.

"On their regular routine duty, the guards co-operated so harmoniously that people would have scarcely known of their existence."

"Oh, Uncle, first I have little engines chugging inside me. Recently I have become some sort of chemistry laboratory and now I have guards!"

"Indeed you do, and these days, it is not like the old way. Enter carbohydrates and the guards have to scramble to their posts and are lucky if they have time off at all!"

"Sorry?" I repeated, looking at him enquiringly.

"So much time spent dealing with the problem of sugar," he said in explanation.

We were standing above the surrounding trees, next to a dumpy but rather charming little monument locally called the pepper-pot and Uncle Wolfi raised his eyes to survey the hazy blue hills in the distance.

"Nowadays . . ." Here Uncle was shaking his head and gazing wistfully at the view, "nowadays we have to call far too often on our regulatory system to sort out the problems we ourselves have created."

For the moment, Uncle seemed to have quite forgotten my existence, so I walked several times round the pepper-pot, glimpsing now the inland hills, now peering into some nearby hazel bushes to see if the squirrels had left any nuts and now appreciating the wide expanse of the bay and the distant sea.

Eventually, I touched Uncle on the elbow:

"Uncle, our regulatory system? Do I have one of those, too?" This was something new and I was interested.

"Ah yes," he said, gathering his thoughts together.

"Next you will be saying I have a computer in my head!"

"Well, in a sense, you do and a very clever one, far cleverer than man has yet invented" Uncle Wolfi was beginning to reply, when I burst in: "I mean, what on earth am I?"

"What are you, Schatz? You are a miracle of life with a highly organised interior! You laugh and sing and study and have a huge back-up system to enable you to do so."

"My Goodness!" I exclaimed.

"A vast back-up system which, unless faulty, you are entirely unaware of. In a vast organisation like the body, part of it has to be devoted to, say, keeping the water balance stable, another to that of salt. And this brings us back to the problem of sugar," said Uncle, though I didn't see quite how.

"You look puzzled, Sparrow. Let us sit down and I'll explain as best I can."

Among a group of nearby rocks, we found a little grassy patch to sit on.

"Part of our bodily organisation is devoted to keeping the level of sugar in the blood stable – that is within certain bounds, just like it is with water and salt.

We have seen how, when it come to carbohydrates, the historic shift from frugality to abundance and especially to overabundance was bound to put great demands on those bits of us that try to keep our bodies running smoothly."

"A shift from 'a sometimes too little' to 'an often too much'," I summarised.

"Quite. From this perspective, you can see the adjustments which the body has to make to this new situation often overtaxes them considerably."

"Quite," I said in my turn.

"One such adjustment, as we have already agreed, is the removal of the resultant and unwanted extra sugar from the bloodstream," continued Uncle.

"But who or what is to see to it?" I asked.

"Indeed, who, let us say, is to give the orders in this new discordant and potentially dangerous situation?

Of course, we do have an overall manager – the big boss, if you like, who knows everything that goes on in the body."

"And all the time?"

"Yes, indeed. However, he does delegate to supervisors and their subordinates a lot of the day-to-day running of the body."

"Is this where the guards come in to defend us?"

"It is. There is, in fact, a whole group of guards working together inside of us who, when 'off duty', see to this day-to day running of our bodies. So let's call them controllers.

They all have their own patch to oversee and their routine duties to perform in their own areas."

"In an emergency, however – and, as you know, removing excess sugar is a task of great urgency – these controller-guards are scrambled into action.

In fact, so crucial is this removal of sugar to our health, that the whole group of controllers is mobilised to achieve this. All need to co-operate with each other and all have to contribute their own skill in one way or another.

I like to think of them as the sugar squad!"

"I like that: sugar squad!" I said appreciatively.

"As we have seen, there are basically two ways for the sugar squad to deal with excess sugar: to store it or to use it.

To work together effectively, a squad needs someone to be in immediate charge. Perhaps not surprisingly, the controller whose job it is to monitor the level of sugar in the bloodstream is given this important position. Let us therefore call him Controller No. 1. Remember he is not the big boss, just in charge of this particular operation."

"He's the Fat Controller!" It was my turn to make a pun, but Uncle didn't get it.

"In more senses than one," said Uncle Wolfi seriously, "as you will see."

"You wonder how the controllers and their associates work together to get rid of extra sugar in the blood?

I shall have to simplify things a little but, in essence, this is what happens: Controller No. 1 instructs the body to convert spare sugar to fat and to put it into storage and, secondly, No. 1 instructs the cells to prefer sugar to make energy rather than to use fat or protein.

Then there is Controller No. 2, one of whose routine jobs is the mobilising of fat for energy. But now, No. 2 is asked by No. 1 to ease up on this job in order to allow sugar to be prioritised as fuel.

There are other controllers, such as Controllers Nos. 3 & 4, who are in charge of making energy from sugar, and these now step up these activities.

 Result: the sugar in the blood is reduced to a safe level."

"Problem solved," said I in admiration.

"Unfortunately, not quite," rejoined Uncle Wolfi. "There are costs to most adjustments and there can be complications, too".

We walked on in order to see if we could get a better glimpse of the shoreline, but were soon back amongst the trees. I scuffled the leaves underfoot.

"So, it is Controller No. 1 which has to make sure our cells with their little engines switch to using sugar instead," I reiterated to check I had understood.

Uncle nodded, "That's one of his jobs, certainly. Now think about this: if the carbohydrate consumption continues to be immoderate, then . . .?"

"Then Controller No. 1 has to go on working overtime to see to this. Well, all of the controllers have to go on overworking."

"Correct. And also?"

"Oh, Uncle, I'm tired with so much thinking!" I complained. "It uses up so much energy," I added to show that I had at least learnt something.

I took a moment to do a cartwheel among the leaves.

"Let's recap. What about your Fat Controller?" asked Uncle with a smile.

"Ah, yes, it's coming back to me".

"And what is our biggest – and potentially huge – storage depot for all that unwanted extra sugar?"

"The fat tissues," I exclaimed, "and Fat Controller No. 1 has a grand time ordering the extra sugar to be changed into fat and sent there."

"Good! Can you work out what happens then?"

"Well, if it's urgent to use up sugar, it's no good allowing fat to be used to make energy, so our bossy Fat Controller puts his foot down and doesn't allow fat to be released from storage at all!" I said proudly.

"Well done! Result: as we have seen, firstly, the body is compelled to run mainly on sugar; secondly, little fat is released; thirdly, ever more fat is stored.

Go and do another bit of your fancy gymnastics, as I have another question for you."

I did as requested.

"Listen carefully, because this next bit is important. Here you have to think of the cumulative effect of the situation. That means the effects added together over time."

Uncle Wolfi always wanted me to understand the mechanics of things.

"I'm listening!"

"You said Controller No.1 would have a grand time ordering unwanted sugar to be turned into fat and sent to the fat tissues.

If the overconsumption of carbohydrates continues over the years, and especially if a sugary or starchy snack is also eaten between meals – for instance accompanying morning tea or afternoon coffee breaks and even at bed-time – then? Can you imagine the result?"

"Ever more fat is stored," I said, reiterating Uncle's own words.

"I'll give you a clue.

Too many sugars and starches eaten
= too much fat created
= too much fat stored by the body
= what?"

"I've got it: VERY FAT PEOPLE!" I shouted, jumping with triumph.

"Precisely: very fat people," confirmed Uncle Wolfi calmly.

"Very fat people," I said again, quite blown over by the idea. "Too many carbohydrates eaten equals too much stored fat equals . . . It seems too simple to be true!"

I couldn't speak for a few minutes.

"Logically, the more carbohydrates eaten, the more sugar there is in the bloodstream to get rid of, and, if not immediately used for energy, the more fat is destined for the fat tissues," repeated Uncle in his turn.

"Obesity can indeed be as simple as that," he added.

"Don't people realise?" I exclaimed, still scarcely believing what I was hearing.

"Lack of energy often accompanies obesity and there are other knock-on effects not so visible", continued Uncle Wolfi, ignoring my incredulity, "but, in essence, that is the process."

"But, but they must know!" I insisted.

"Of course, it is known! Or at least the knowledge is available," muttered Uncle Wolfi, author of many books.

"So why do they go on telling us that we should eat so much carbohydrate?"

"Perhaps, having denigrated what they see as the over consumption of fat and protein, they are reluctant to denounce the overconsumption of carbohydrate, lest people feel there is nothing safe left to eat?" replied Uncle sardonically.

"I spot a problem, Uncle Wolfi," I said. "If people eat lots of carbohydrate, it can make them fat. But if people eat lots of fat as well, surely it can make them even fatter?"

"It's a good point, Spatz. Can you spot why this might be so?" asked Uncle.

"Well, Controller No. 1 stops access to body fat when too many carbohydrates are eaten. It is like having a food cupboard where you can put items in but then the door is locked and you can't get anything out again. So I presume that, as the door stays locked, extra fat from fat can be added to the cupboard but not retrieved? So people do get even fatter!"

"You are right enough and this point often leads to wrong thinking. It leads to people being then advised either to cut down on their intake of both fat and carbohydrate – as though both were equally at fault – or else to cut down on fat, rather than carbohydrate, which is quite the wrong way round.

Amongst other reasons we need fat is, as you well know . . ."

"Because energy has to come from somewhere!" I said, quoting one of Uncle's regular sayings.

"What we always have to remember is that it is not fat per se that makes us fat – not the fat we eat, anyway," commented Uncle Wolfi, "as it does not disturb our controllers in the same way."

Fat does not disturb our controllers in the same way, I repeated to myself. Now that was something to think about!

"Ironically," continued Uncle, "Eating fat can help you, not put on, but lose body fat!" Uncle was losing me again. "In fact, I feel that the current level of obesity in our society is wholly preventable, but there is one important proviso. . ."

"One important proviso," I echoed. That rang a bell.

"That we don't eat too many carbohydrates!" we chorused in unison and we both laughed together.

"So, Uncle Wolfi to sum up," I said, growing serious again, "getting fat, even very fat, is one of the costs of having to remove so much sugar from the blood. In turn, having so much sugar in the blood is one of the costs of eating so much starchy food in the first place, not to mention sugary food.

And none of this would happen if we had stuck to seal meat! Hey, ho!" I concluded and leap-frogged over one of the rocks

17 DOWNHILL

Uncle Wolfi stood up and, having a good stretch of his arms, looked around again with appreciation:

"What a view! You do live in a lovely place, yet so unlike my Austrian mountains."

"I love it," I said, glancing up at the seagulls circling overhead. "There is a place where water drips through the limestone rock and it comes out very pure. People make their beer with it. And there is an apple tree a hundred years old!"

Uncle smiled at my enthusiasm.

"But your train, Uncle," I said. "We ought to be getting back."

"Indeed, we ought," agreed Uncle looking at his watch. "We can continue our conversation on the way, can't we."

With one last look at the scenery, we left the pepper-pot and retraced our steps through the wood towards home.

"I said that obesity can be as simple as that, and it can. But, you know, things are seldom as simple as one thinks or as one might like them to be!

For instance, if you come from generations of overeaters of carbohydrate or even just have, say, overweight parents, things often don't run as smoothly as they might otherwise.

I have noticed, too, that trouble seems to get earlier by the generation, and especially since this craze for reducing even traditional fats." Here Uncle Wolfi sighed.

I sighed, too, at that ominous word 'trouble'.

"Even so, added Uncle, "with remedial action, problems are not inevitable. You look wistful, Sparrow! What is it?"

"Well, I thought the controllers were supposed to be on our side and would try to do the best for us at all times, yet they make us fat and the rest of it!" I said, protesting slightly at their seeming dereliction of duty.

"There is an answer to that, Sparrow. You see, there is short-term wisdom and long-term wisdom.

The body has to react with short-term wisdom, especially when safeguarding the sugar levels in the bloodstream, and therefore cannot at the same time act in a way which might prevent problems later on, such as might stem from obesity."

"I can see that, yes, in that case the body is still on our side," I conceded reluctantly.

"So where did we get up to? Ah, yes, to store or to use: the question of what to do with any extraneous sugar in the bloodstream.

We have already spoken of the storage of the excess as fat, and that is certainly one way, shall we say, that we get out of balance, one response to the stress of too many carbohydrates, one manifestation of the carbohydrate effect.

There is another scenario, which I have never fully understood", said Uncle, "and in which the use of sugar to make energy seems to predominate over its storage as fat."

"So lots and lots of energy?" I queried.

"I'm talking of people who are very thin. Perhaps it is the other side of the coin, as it were."

"Fattypuffs and thinifers", I said. Uncle looked blank.

"Patapouf et filifer," I added in my best French accent. A smile crept over Uncle Wolfi's face.

"Maurois? André? The two brothers always fighting, the one short and fat and the other tall and very thin and ever restless?

Thin, nervous and ever on the go," reflected Uncle Wolfi. "I remember I was like that once, despite the Austrian pastries!"

"And look at me and my biscuits and cake! Just the same!" I exclaimed and then paused.

"Uncle Wolfi, my problem" I said at length, "Is that, in the book, the podgy one was always eating whereas the skinny one hardly ate at all.

I can see that if you hardly eat anything you will be half starved, and you'll get very thin. But I've got friends who are thinifers who never stop eating – and they are always eating lots of carbohydrates just like the fattypuffs."

"Of course, apart from serious illness, there are many reasons why people get so thin," said my cautious Uncle, the doctor of long experience.

"Maybe they don't have enough traditional fats in their diet?" I suggested.

"Very probably! Or enough protein, come to that!"

"So we skinifers eat carbohydrates by the bun load but we don't seem to put on fat though, according to what you said before we ought to.

And, Uncle, we skinny people are buzzing with energy and consumed in mega-activity. Have you noticed how we seem to get faster and faster?" I asked, speaking faster and faster myself and beginning to jump up and down with excitement.

"Consumed is an interesting word!" commented Uncle.

"But do you think we just can't stop burning sugar?" I queried, rushing at the subject. "Or is it that we have so much sugar to burn that we have to be always on the go? Or is it that we just can't make fat, and so have to burn more and more sugar?" adding, a bit more meekly, "It's just a thought, Uncle Wolfi."

"We don't exactly <u>burn</u> sugar, Schatz," commented Uncle slowly. "And yes, the balance between controllers is certainly involved. Our modern diet, as I said, does tend to exact a constant over-exertion from all the various controllers through continual need for their services."

"Uncle Wolfi, you said that the controllers in charge of making energy from sugar step up their work when we need to get rid of sugar", I persisted. "Aren't these the very controllers that help us in emergency when running from polar bears?"

"They would be helping, certainly."

"So if we needed to create more and more energy, couldn't we just get thinner and thinner and more and more nervy, like we get fatter and fatter and become couch potatoes from storing fat?"

I had visions of eventual implosion or explosion.

"Yes, that is a potential problem, though naturally it is not as straightforward as that. Let us call it a tendency. The body has lots of ways of steadying this process, so don't go frightening yourself!"

"But there are such a lot of very thin people around as well as a lot of very fat ones!" I protested. "Do you think one of the energy controllers goes on overdrive and so overdoes it?"

"It is certainly a possibility. There is an important balance to be kept, you are quite right there and, sadly, things can get out of hand."

"You see, both underweight and overweight are states of disequilibrium – imbalance, if you like", continued Uncle.

131

"Like a swing of the pendulum – a plus or a minus, but either way not staying in the middle", I mused.

Uncle smiled: "The bit I can't quite figure out is exactly what it is that triggers the pendulum to swing one way or the other. I've often thought about this."

"I seem to be swinging to the minus", I said gloomily.

"Oh, you are not that thin, Sparrow!" added Uncle Wolfi comfortingly.

"Oh yes, I am. But you, Uncle, you don't seem to be either podgy or skinny, but tall and upright – and calm, too!"

"But then maybe I know the secret, don't you think?" said Uncle Wolfi with that old twinkle in his eyes.

"Therefore, Uncle Wolfi," I said, continuing my quest for understanding, "obesity and over-thinness could both, in fact, come from eating too many carbohydrates!"

"As I said, there are a lot of things which can influence our weight. You see it is not just what you eat but how well you digest and absorb the food, also how the body uses it.

Nevertheless, over the years I have seen many people, both fat and thin, regain their proper figures by sticking to my diet, it is true.

I've also shown clinically that, when carbohydrates are sufficiently reduced, this calms the overactivity of all the major controllers – except that the previously suppressed Controller No. 2 is stimulated. Remember Controller No. 2?

So you have a point, Sparrow, and an important one!"

"And people calm down and are much more peaceful and less hungry?" I said, pursuing the point.

"Yes, indeed", confirmed Uncle. "And the point about No. 2 no longer being suppressed is important for several reasons.

You see, it is not just that it encourages fat to be used for fuel but, being a builder of tissue, it helps the health and so efficiency of those bits of the body that fight infection."

"So less colds and flu?"

"Much more resistant to all sorts of infections," said Uncle. "Perhaps surprisingly, my diet has also proven helpful to those who are very thin, who eat far too little and who seem reluctant to eat at all."

"And peck at their food like little birds? I know someone at school like that," I commented.

Uncle's face showed he agreed. "What I can say is that these people do well on the diet: they fill out, become sturdier and get an appetite for food once more.

It is all a question of balance, as I said, and disequilibrium shows itself in being either too lethargic or too energetic . . ."

"Too fast or too slow, too nervy or too placid, too overexcited or too dull, too fat or too thin, too light or too heavy and so on?" I added with enthusiasm.

"All of which," concluded Uncle Wolfi, nodding slowly, "can be manifestations of the carbohydrate effect, that is they could all be part of the price we are paying for us choosing to make carbohydrate our primary fuel."

18 A WORKING COMPROMISE

"Uncle Wolfi, I do admire you and I know you are very special, but . . ."

"But?" prompted Uncle, one eyebrow raised.

"But you must admit that not everyone stuffs themselves with carbohydrate, nor do they eat as little carbohydrate as you appear to do or would probably recommend.

For example, there are plenty of people who are neither podgy nor skinny and who seem healthy enough."

"I freely admit it," said Uncle. "Remember we have been looking at extremes, that is the many and very varied end results of far too high an intake of carbohydrate.

I agree that there are people who eat moderately – that is their carbohydrate consumption is not as low as I myself think ideal – yet who are apparently healthy and of good physique."

"So, Uncle, the picture is not all gloom and doom. I'm glad of that. I'd love to know how that works, though."

"Ah, now that is interesting, and a pattern seen so frequently that it is nowadays described as the norm."

"I'll tell you about it, Sparrow. Now think controllers!" ordered Uncle Wolfi.

"I'm thinking controllers," I said touching my pretend cap.

"If consumption of carbohydrates is not too high – and, as I said, for many people who eat modestly this is still the case – then Controller No. 1 rules the roost for a couple of hours after a meal, sorting out the rise in blood sugar that follows eating.

After that, No. 1 steps down, allowing Controller No. 2 not only to get on with his other jobs better, such as seeing to the growth, repair and renewal of tissues, but also to order fat to be used for fuel once more. This includes the fat made from the modest amount of carbohydrate eaten."

"A sort of working compromise between then and now, between the old way and the new way?" I put in.

"Yes, if you like, and this is usually the way for people with moderate appetites. For some people, this arrangement can go on fairly unproblematically for years, occasionally lifelong.

As a result, reasonable health and normal weight can be maintained, especially in those who are active, have a sound constitution, good heredity and, as I said, who don't overeat generally. Of course, healthy strong controllers help!"

"A tall order!" I mused, "but good news for some."

"Good news for some, certainly."

"If it works, why isn't it your way, Uncle Wolfi? Surely, it can't just be your penchant for evolutionary history!"

"No, Schatz, not that!" said Uncle laughing. "Why isn't it my way? Well, because it doesn't work for everyone.

Remember what I just said about heredity! Remember, too, about more thorough measures being sometimes needed for the sick than for the healthy.

Now think how ill I was all those years ago when I was scarcely able to follow my profession anymore. I needed both to get well and then stay well. For me, a compromise solution was not an option. Hence I needed my low carbohydrate diet!"

"Too many years on too many sugars and starches!" I concluded. Uncle merely nodded.

"Sadly, there are many people who have also spent too many years on too many sugars and starches and for them, too, my low carbohydrate might be the only way to stay well. Or maybe there are several members of your family – say, your aunt, grandpa and great-grandma - who suffer or suffered from terrible headaches like I did, and especially if they ate certain foods: this does not mean you will inevitably suffer from these headaches. However, you may have inherited a susceptibility to such a condition and might find that you, too, thrive better if you not only go steady on those foods but also eat sugars and starches in moderation. It is good to be aware of these things."

By now, we were back on the road that led to our house. I knew Mum would have the kettle on and the tea things ready. Still we talked on.

"Does this answer your question about our main source of energy, Sparrow?"

I hesitated: "So you think that, nowadays, we have got the wrong end of the stick in thinking sugar to be a better internal fuel than fat for general purposes – or even just for muscles?

"I do indeed!"

"And that it is folly to think that we can eat a lot of sugar and starch, put on a lot of body fat and then sit around in the hope that it will burn off again when we next go to the gym or for a long walk?

Surely, in that case the muscles will still need to burn sugar rather than fat?"

"Indeed they will. And why does this matter? Can you put it in a nutshell, Sparrow?"

"Something about using sugar as our main fuel putting the body in a state of constant emergency, thereby exhausting our controllers with overwork. And this is followed by all sorts of consequences, some minor and some dire."

"Not bad! You have been taking it in. Well done!"

"Let me recap," suggested Uncle. "Now, in your country and mine, there is plenty of choice as to what we can eat.

For those who choose to eat little carbohydrate, the main dietary source of energy is likely to be fat. I know it is so for me. And therefore the main internal source of energy is also likely to be fat."

"In our little cell engines only, this time, not the cell spaces?"

"Yes, Sparrow, only in the little cell engines."

"When people eat slightly more carbohydrate, then carbohydrate may or may not form the main dietary source of energy.

The bodies of these people run, not exactly on half and half, but their cells alternate between using mainly sugar and using mainly fat to make energy. For many people, this can work fairly comfortably, as you know."

"The working compromise?"

"Exactly so!" confirmed Uncle Wolfi.

"However", continued my knowledgeable but scary Uncle, "once the consumption of carbohydrate becomes, shall we say, immoderate, then carbohydrate becomes not only our main dietary source of energy but also our main source of energy at cell level.

This is because, as I've already explained, to save our very lives the 'burning' of excess sugar as fuel has to take priority over the use of fat – the body has no choice in the matter."

So you see," concluded Uncle Wolfi, "the fact of the matter is simply this: the more carbohydrate we eat – and by 'more', I am talking not of percentages but of the actual amount of sugars and starches eaten – the more carbohydrate actually does become our main source of energy."

"Oh Uncle," I said, and fell silent.

I knew he was right.

Mum was at the door to meet us:

"Come on you two. Tea is ready and time is running out."

Uncle, ever polite, greeted Mum and thanked her for the tea. Then, as soon as he sat down, off he went again:

"I am sorry to say that this new reality is rapidly becoming the norm in everyday life."

"For the compromise was only a compromise. Once carbohydrates become the main source of our energy, the already precarious balance is firmly tipped to the wrong side," I contributed.

"Yes, and confusion results and the thin line between truth and error is crossed.

Importantly, the link with our past is broken: any idea as to what ought to be our main internal energy source according to our origin as a species or according to the inherent design of our bodies – and so any notion as to best practice – is lost."

Uncle Wolfi shook his head sadly and sighed as he thought of this broken link with our past and with what he referred to as our inherent design.

"You see, it may be true that, for many if not most people, carbohydrate has become their main internal source of energy, but – and this is a big but . . ."

Then soft-spoken Uncle Wolfi stopped mid-sentence and became slower and more emphatic, tapping his knee every few words to give more weight to them.

"But THIS, as I said before, does NOT IMPLY that CARBOHYDRATE is therefore the NATURAL and most health-promoting MAIN SOURCE OF FUEL for us humans. That is an ERROR!

Carbohydrate, as I also told you before, is NOT even our MOST EFFICIENT fuel! To see carbohydrate as the MOST DESIRABLE source of energy AT CELL LEVEL is very definitely an ERROR, an error which too often leads to WIDESPREAD and DISASTROUS CONSEQUENCES for our HEALTH and our WELLBEING.

And there you have it!"

Here Uncle looked at his watch again and then at me.

"Worry not, niece of mine," he said gently. "Just always remember that WE OURSELVES DO HAVE A CHOICE IN THIS MATTER."

It was time for Uncle Wolfi to get himself ready to depart. He gathered his few things together and Mum brought his coat. As he was putting it on, he turned to me:

"Sparrow, now that you are beginning to 'get my drift', as you put it, would you consider being useful to me?

Writing English I find so much more difficult than speaking it and I want to write an article or two about my work while I'm in London.

I am also thinking of working on a summary of Leben ohne Brot in English. Naturally, I'll do all the notes and technical terms – and there won't be words like 'narky', 'scuppered' or 'probs'.

If I make notes, would you be kind enough to write it out in good English? I know you are capable. I would be so pleased if you would."

"I'll try, Uncle Wolfi, I'll try," I said, honoured as well as overawed by the request.

"Good, good!" responded Uncle in satisfaction.

"I hear the taxi," I said, jumping up.

We all said our farewells and in no time at all, Uncle Wolfi was off and away.

PART III

DOING A WOLFI

17 HOMEWORK

To be worthy of Uncle Wolfi's trust, I had plenty of homework to do. The week after his visit, Uncle sent me a copy of what he referred to as his 'red book', as the English translation of his book had a red cover.

Over the years, Uncle had added lots of extra bits to his main book, Leben ohne Brot. It had reached its ninth edition before being translated.

But here it was in English, Dismantling a Myth: the Role of Fat and Carbohydrates in our Diet, my very own red book.

Full of curiosity, I started reading. In it, Uncle began by saying that there had been doctors before him who had had similar ideas about diet.

Even at the time of his 'awakening' some fifty years ago, there was a doctor, very high up in the medical profession in America, who was putting his patients on a diet more extreme than Uncle's.

Meat, meat fat and coffee were allowed, which seemed very much like what Stef ate during his experimental year in New York except that, in practice, this particular doctor permitted the occasional vegetable.

Uncle, I knew, was far more liberal than that, for I hadn't forgotten those delicious tiny delicacies I had eaten for dessert at his home in Austria as a child.

In his red book, Uncle Wolfi tells the story of how he came to connect the eating of carbohydrates, and especially the overeating of them, with various bodily upsets and how this changed his ideas on medicine.

Looking at the impressive range of ailments he appeared to have treated – or even just at the chapter headings – gave me an inkling of what Uncle Wolfi was driving at when I had formerly quizzed him about the effects of excess carbohydrate and he had summed it up in the one word: 'trouble'.

It was quite early on in his work as a doctor that Uncle had grown fascinated by problems to do with the internal regulation of our bodies and in particular the interplay between different disturbances.

In one foreword, it said that Uncle Wolfi was one of the first people to spot certain links in this area, especially the sort of links between the upsettable regulators which he had started explaining to me.

I knew it was for the sake of my young age that Uncle had called these regulators 'controllers'. Since my main interest was in how things operated, I still used this term.

Uncle Wolfi did make a real attempt to make this book intelligible to interested people like me who weren't medics.

I liked, for example, the way he described living on our present mixed diet as rather like the experience of driving a sports car on inferior, regular petrol which was not quite suitable, as compared to the delightfully smooth run driving such a car on super.

Not that I had ever even ridden in a sports car, but this appealed to my imagination!

I liked, too, the way that, even in his red book, Uncle talked about the 'sugar squad' when referring to the group of controllers responsible for keeping the level of blood sugar within safe bounds. So I found that it was not just for me that he did this.

However, Uncle wrote not just for lay people but also with his fellow doctors in mind.

Accordingly, the book was quite hard-going and I confess that a lot of it was beyond me as yet. The complicated names and technical phrases dazzled me. The subtitle of his later editions of *Leben ohne Brot,* that is *Die wissenschaftlichen Grundlagen der kohlenhydratarmen Ernährung* – the scientific foundation of low carbohydrate nutrition, or was it the fundamental principles? – should have warned me!

And there were so many diseases! Perhaps I was not old enough to cope with thinking about all those bits of people that can go wrong?

I therefore contented myself with trying to understand from the red book a bit more about the basic processes, which Uncle and I had been discussing.

I was reminded that, just as in prehistoric times, our body still worked as a whole and that our health depended on every part of the body co-operating in a co-ordinated effort.

I learnt that the special controllers, which Uncle Wolfi took such an interest in, had their seats in the various glands in question, each having its own task or tasks to perform yet all needing to pull together.

Yes, the controllers did work under a big boss and this was situated in the brain and all of them sent their instructions for various bodily processes straight into the bloodstream. Controller No. 1, as Uncle had said to me, had the power to give orders to the other squad members in the event of a blood sugar emergency.

It was interesting to read more on how the controllers shared and adjusted to each other's workloads.

I had already seen that if one controller was called on to do more than usual, then another might have to do less to make this possible, and how sometimes there needed to be a particular type of teamwork for them to achieve the same goal.

I had also seen that if you upset one controller too much, then this might upset the others in a sort of chain reaction.

But now I learned that it wasn't just the controllers that suffered: there were layer upon layer of related activities going on inside us that were also affected.

Moreover, this chain of knock-on effects could go on and on, until there were bodily disturbances that were so far removed from the beginning of the chain that the original source of any disturbance was lost to view, and so difficult to pin down.

Phew! Just as Uncle had pointed out when we were together!

It all made a sort of sense to me, but it didn't make it any clearer why someone's corns disappeared if they ate fewer carbohydrates!

I suppose one answer might be that, as Uncle had said, skin quality improved. But then what had skin quality to do with eating sugars and starches? Ah – a glimmer of light!

Was it that eating less carbohydrate imposed less restriction on the controller in charge of skin quality?

This had to be Controller No. 2. For Uncle seemed to think that being told to go easy on arranging fat to be fetched from the fat cells affected No. 2's ability to perform its other duties, including the fighting of infection and the renewal of tissue.

But would neglected skin renewal and repair make you more liable to corns? It had to be possible and Uncle Wolfi had said his skin became more resilient and chafed less.

This was getting exciting.

In the wake of this thought, I began to better understand why, with the intake of carbohydrate much reduced, there was a chance for positive collaboration between the controllers in keeping our body strong and healthy.

With his work no longer hampered by Controller No. 1, Controller No. 2 could now see to the ongoing work of renewal and repair. With the cells again free to choose the fuel to suit the purpose in hand, whether fat, carbohydrate or protein, No. 2 could instruct the release of any necessary fat.

In effect, by restricting carbohydrate, the key was restored to the previously locked food cupboard.

Co-operation was certainly more constructive than opposition! Was this the sort of thing hinted at by Uncle's comment about harmony prevailing only if . . .?

However, it turned out that unlocking the food cupboard was not always so simple and that changes consequent on eating carbohydrate were not always easy to reverse.

Overeating carbohydrates might cause a great accumulation of body fat, for instance, and this in itself led to alterations in the balance of controller activity.

Uncle said in his red book that such changes could sometimes assume an independent nature and so might persist even after carbohydrates had been curtailed.

Uncle Wolfi did not say, I noticed, that it was therefore not worth trying to restrict carbohydrates, just that this may limit or delay success in, say, slimming.

But back to carbohydrate overload. One thing I couldn't figure out was the bit about the 'working compromise'.

It was fine for Controllers No. 1 and No. 2 to swap places for two hours or so after a meal and, yes, the compromise would work if we ate carbohydrates modestly.

But even if we ate sweet and stodgy things all day and so blocked access to fat all day, surely there were still eight hours or so left during the night for Controller No. 2 to get busy?

I asked Uncle Wolfi, who said something about bodies getting into a habitual way of doing things and that, if things had got that bad, eight hours weren't long enough to make the switch to a different fuel.

Uncle then painted a gruesome picture of us consuming protein from our own body tissues to provide the necessary sugar, just like it had to do during, say, a famine.

And there was something even more gruesome about plugging the gaps in the damaged tissues with fat.

It sounded dire. But what did 'things getting that bad' mean in practice? I searched in my other books. Except in cases of real starvation, I could not find out. Nor could I discover how much carbohydrate it would take to get there.

Talking of disturbances and things getting bad, I thought for a moment of the poor cells!

I knew that millions if not trillions of our cells stored minute amounts of starch, fat and protein to provide energy, and that they didn't want much sugar in the first place.

So I could imagine how, when asked to take in ever more sugar, there has to come a time when the cells are full to the gunwales of sugar and say 'enough is enough': they sulk, resist the commands from outside (defying Controller No. 1) and shut their gates. Cells would have to have been very provoked over a long period of time to behave like that, I thought.

147

As for the controllers getting cantankerous, imagine being a guard and having to be constantly on emergency duty!

True, No. 1's job was to be always on duty, always present in the bloodstream checking sugar levels and to be around after each mealtime as well as getting on happily with other tasks.

That was fine and normal and No. 1 obligingly saw to the odd bit of excess sugar now and then, or even several times a day, without making too much fuss.

However, to be always on emergency duty?

I managed to get a quick word with Uncle on the phone.

"Oh, Uncle, this business of being always on emergency duty: it takes the biscuit!"

"Biscuits again, Sparrow, surely not!" remonstrated Uncle.

"It's only an expression, Uncle Wolfi. What I mean is that being on permanent call-out is ridiculous. It is too much to demand. Such service could definitely not be sustained. How can the controllers possibly keep it up?"

"The situation is just as I said, Spatz. They have no time off because they are too busy dealing with the problem of sugar!'

"But Uncle, what then?"

"Ah, that is the next question for you to look into! Good luck with it. Must go!"

I did look into the question of 'what then?' and I found that increasing the size of the guard did not long suffice.

Over-demanded Controller No. 1 soon started thinking: 'I know what is coming – my owner always has toast and marmalade for breakfast and she has sugar with her coffee.

There will be constant other starches and sugars coming in throughout the day and evening, too – so forget all this fine

148

tuning, I'll just throw out a generous handful of instructions as to getting rid of extraneous sugar. It's sure to cover the need.'

Cover the need it does, but proves over-generous and too many instructions are sent out.

The result of this largesse is that too much blood sugar is removed. Rather than a surplus, there is now too little sugar in the bloodstream and the owner herself feels wobbly, anxious and irritable and cantankerous!

Soon the controllers from the sugar squad whose job it was to created energy rush in to help: Controllers Nos. 3 and 4 initiate feelings of hunger and mobilise sugar from anywhere they can get it – from the small stores of starch in the muscles and liver or creating it from waste proteins.

If really necessary, they indulge in that horrid process that I mentioned before, that is of ordering sugar to be created from protein belonging to their own body tissues.

Between them, the controllers nevertheless do a good job in topping up the sugar level again.

Now here lies the main difficulty – the 'generous handful of instructions' provided by Controller No. 1 becomes habitual. It isn't long, therefore, before all the involved controllers become extra over-worked.

The owner now feels as though she were living on a roller coaster.

Not good, not good at all.

So this was why, when I wanted to eat again half an hour after a meal, Uncle had accused me of having false hunger?

My 'hunger' was real in the sense of the blood's immediate need for sugar, but this was the consequence, not of having too little to eat, but rather of my having had too much of, well, need I say what?

It's true I felt wobbly and also irritable, sometimes fearful, sometimes tearful. Eating a sweetie would put that right for a while, until the next time, that is.

And it was always difficult to stop eating biscuits. I would take one, and then find I had finished the whole packet. It was the same with chocolate. Oh dear!

But this wasn't all, as I found out when I delved back into my red book.

Apparently, if this condition lasts too long, Controller No. 1 gradually becomes more and more exhausted and can't hack it any more: fewer and fewer instructions are sent out and so sugar mounts in the bloodstream unchecked.

The owner now has a recognised ailment. Uncle said that, at this stage, it was often still possible to live safely and healthily by keeping to his way of eating. This he knew from his many years of experience working as a doctor.

All this did make sense, I thought.

If you ate few enough carbohydrates, this had to mean there was no excess sugar in the blood. Then there would no longer be any call on Controller No. 1 for continuous emergency duty, nor call on any of the other Controllers, as Uncle Wolfi's diet offered cells a fuel more suited to their purpose. I could imagine how gratefully Controller No. 1 and co would return to regular duties, now that overtime was no longer necessary.

Surely, this might stop all those ill effects from all those various disturbances in all those different parts of the body and in the future, too, I wondered?

Yet if the overload of carbohydrate continued and so the need for overtime, the person in question has to be supplied by doctors with a stand-in from outside the body to assist her own over-wearied Controller No. 1.

She then feels better in herself and can carry on eating more or less the same way as before.

However – and this is important– if she does not mend her ways and reduce her sugars and starches, this does not stop the cells eventually resisting and going on strike. But who thinks: 'Poor cells, you've had more than enough sugar already, so to help me you are shutting your gates'? No, this gate-shutting is seen as another illness, which is given its own name and for which drugs are developed to force the cells to open their gates to take in even more sugar!

Nor does it prevent all the other controllers being adversely affected, and particularly No. 2, so important for tissue quality.

Result: all sorts of other trouble, some very serious and much of it avoidable!

Good old Uncle Wolfi, he must have saved his patients from so much suffering. I was proud of him.

I told Mum of all I had read and she became very serious, then said: "Well, you have to hand it to the old boy!"

"What, my chocolate?" I said, alarmed.

"No, silly, can't you see he's trying, after his own fashion, to give you a wake-up call?"

"I . . . um . . . well . . . but . . ." is all I could manage.

I looked at Mum, but Mum, lapsing into deep thought, just muttered: "I wonder, I just wonder."

18 DECISION TIME

Mum and I did a lot of wondering. About a week later we were having a meal together and were reflecting on Uncle Wolfi's last visit.

"I thought Uncle was very considerate in not bogging us down with the long names of all those internal bits and pieces. I've got enough to learn at school," I grumbled, adding, "and I was thankful he didn't talk about all those awful ailments which he seems to treat so successfully. There were more than enough in his book!"

"You mean those he so charmingly refers to as the 'civilisatory diseases'?"

"Yes, and Mum, you ought to have another look at the red book – the list is awesome!"

"I wish you would not use that term, dear!"

"Oh, Mum, but it does seem Uncle has found a wonderful tool for healing, don't you think?"

"I believe so," she said, "judging by my own very limited experience, anyway. Praise be, we do not need him to treat us for any of his 'awful ailments', as you call them."

Not yet, I thought inwardly.

"But perhaps proper instructions as to his diet, we do require," she added.

I looked at Mum. What did she mean by 'we do require'? Had she made up her mind? Would she take the plunge?

"I could give Uncle a ring and ask his advice, maybe," I said cautiously.

"No, I'll give the old boy a bell myself."

She called him 'the old boy' as often as he called me Sparrow.

"I think we should give it a try," said Mum mildly. She looked at me: "don't you agree?"

"I suppose I agree," I said, heavy-hearted, with visions of all sorts of goodies disappearing from the shelves of the fridge and a bleak freezer stocked with reindeer meat. "Yes, Mum, if Uncle says I ought, I'll give it a go," I said reluctantly.

Uncle was duly phoned. The feedback I got was that he was delighted and wished us every success with it.

As Mum was 'of a certain age' it would be better for her to start slowly, say take several months in cutting down to his magic amount, but that I, a teenager, could probably cut down straight away.

"You don't think I'm going to sit here fiddling with my fish fingers while you scoff all the chips do you?" I said, testily.

"The old boy did suggest it was always easier if another member of the household was also doing it – and at the same rate – he said it preserved domestic harmony!" she smiled, knowingly.

I grimaced, but Mum ignored me and went on.

"And I was to make sure I did not cut down fat as well as carbohydrate which, he said, was where a lot of people went wrong. I told him to have no fear – it would be a blessed relief not to have to worry any more about cutting down fat.

I said I was already eating a little more fat and that some days I found I wanted more than others. He said that was how it should be and that, provided you chose natural fats and cut down the carbohydrates enough, the body regulated its own appetite for them – too little and you wanted more, too much and you felt nauseous."

"Uncle is right," I put in, "you couldn't eat a whole packet of butter in one go, could you!"

I grinned at my own cleverness, and added: "But if the meat is dry, a little butter is good." I had seen Uncle Wolfi do this.

"The good news," said Mum, "is that on this diet the need for calories also regulates itself, so we can throw out altogether any thought of counting calories – a red herring, according to your Uncle Wolfi."

"Why's that, Mum?"

"Something about fat not disturbing the body's regulators in the same way. You must ask him yourself what that means."

"Oh, it will be Controller No. 1 again," I said half to myself.

"Controller No. 1" queried Mum.

"Controller No. 1 gets very upset when we eat too many carbohydrates, whereas he doesn't even blink when it is fat," I explained without making anything clearer.

Mum merely shook her head.

"QED: it is carbs not calories that count!" I concluded.

"Did Uncle mention chickens?" I asked on a sudden impulse, for there was something at the back of my mind.

"Well, yes he did. He said he let his chickens choose for themselves the amount of food they ate. Some had low-fat feed with a lot of carbohydrate, others had more fat and little carbohydrate. It was noticed that the high carbohydrate lot always came running for more."

Sounds familiar, I thought!

"It was found that the calorie intake was far higher in those Wolfgang fed with a high carbohydrate feed than those that had little carbohydrate and more fat in their feed," finished Mum.

"Yes, and then his friend did nearly the same experiment but kept calories equal. Result? The hens eating low fat and which got their calories mainly from carbohydrate – mostly from grain – got ill, whereas the ones eating few carbos, no grain and more fat stayed healthy!" I added.

"Got ill from what?" asked Mum.

"Oh some long word to do with arteries or something."

Mum fell silent, thinking.

"And did you know, mum, that hens only lay so many eggs because of the way we feed them? I bet you didn't!

I remember Uncle saying that there was something in grain that upset their reproductive systems and made them lay far more eggs than was natural for a bird.

Whether it was the carbohydrate in the grain or something else, he didn't say."

Mum looked even more thoughtful.

"And I said did it upset ours, too? I gathered that it might, but he was reluctant to answer, saying I would learn about that later. Only I haven't learnt yet!"

"Your Uncle did say it would 'do the little one good'."

Little one! I could learn to drive in a couple of years! I was almost adult, I thought angrily. But then, he was such an old man himself I had to forgive him.

Moreover, just maybe, this was part of his answer?"

"So you and I, Mum, are to cut down carbohydrates and to be careful not to cut down fats as well. That's clear!

But Mum, did he say how far I, myself, was to cut down the carbs in order to 'do me good'?"

"Well, yes, he said that it would be best if you aimed at reducing to about 72 g of carbohydrate daily and that I could perhaps reduce a little less."

Now that rang a bell. Seventy-two grams – I had seen that figure often enough in the red book.

"But why 72 g" queried Mum, "and why so precise?"

"According to Uncle Wolfi, people find it helpful to have a precise target to aim at, even if in reality the amount can only be approximate. It sort of makes sense, for he says that even apples will vary in their carbohydrate content."

"Yes, I can see that," said Mum, "but why the 72 g?"

"That was because, early on when Uncle worked in a rural area, he had a lot of fat young kids under his care, whose Controller No. 1 used to go a bit berserk with overactivity.

Uncle says that he measured their blood sugar levels and it seems that 72 g was the maximum level of carbohydrate they could tolerate daily without this happening!"

Mum looked at me bemused.

"But wait until you hear the next bit! Get this: before the war, Uncle used to work in a hospital where there was a clinic for treating blood sugar problems of a different type – where Controller No. 1 gets worn out, I think.

Anyway, the clinic was in Vienna, and Uncle had a chance to observe what happened there. Do you know what?

To keep the sugar level stable in these patients, the clinic also found that 72 g was the maximum level of carbohydrate tolerated! Uncle said for the common type of this condition it was very effective.

In those days, they didn't have proper drugs and there was no high-tech equipment, so they had to observe their patients closely over many years. They then relied on practical measures such as diet to control the condition.

So that is what they did."

"Apparently", I continued: "apart from having limits on their carbohydrate consumption, the patients had a free choice as to the amount of fat and protein they could eat. Fat was certainly not denied to them nor, according to Uncle, even restricted.

Uncle said that energy had to come from somewhere, so I suppose it was OK for patients to eat as much fat as they liked.

What fry-ups they could have! Just imagine!"

Mum pulled a slightly impatient face at my last suggestion.

"You haven't heard the best bit yet," said I.

"Go on," encouraged Mum.

"Well, you know about the horrid things that can happen to people's eyesight. Uncle said not only was the diet effective but it even prevented – let me get Uncle's words right – 'the highly distressing complications to the eyes and blood vessels'.

And I said was it really true about preventing complications? And Uncle said:

'Oh yes, prevented and often healed, but patients obviously had to be willing to co-operate and to stick to the diet in the long term. Most did and benefited accordingly.'"

"That's amazing, and so different from nowadays!" said Mum, thinking of the tough time one of her cousins had gone through recently.

"But what I can't understand," continued Mum, "is why Wolfgang didn't stick to that Vienna diet for ever after. What's the point of rediscovering something you already know!"

"I asked him the same question! The truth is, I don't think Uncle had really cottoned on to low carbs in those days."

"And what did the old boy actually say?"

157

"Talking of the clinic's success in helping its patients by stabilising their blood sugar, he said:

'I did not realise how fundamental such stability was to the progression or otherwise of many other conditions, nor did I realise how crucial it was for our health in general not to upset our internal regulatory mechanisms too much.'

How's that for a demo of Uncle's immaculate English?"

"I sometimes wish you would follow his good example, Sparrow! I myself think 'carbs', 'carbos' and 'carbohydrates' are all ugly words, whichever way you say them," said Mum. "It reminds me of chemistry lessons! I vote we stick to 'sugars and starches', don't you?"

"Not easy," I replied sagely. "To 'do a Wolfi' properly, we have to learn about quantities, so we can't escape the C word entirely."

"A great pity, such horrid words and at mealtimes, too," was Mum's rejoinder, "and all that weighing and measuring we'll have to do! And adding up all those grams!"

"Don't worry, Mum, there is a way," I announced. "Luckily for us, Uncle has a wonderfully simple way of calculating."

"Well?" challenged Mum.

"Well, Uncle Wolfi uses bread units," I announced.

Uncle Wolfi had told me that he had got acquainted with the bread unit during his time in Vienna.

"Bread units?" queried Mum.

"Yes, each unit has 12 grams of carbohydrate. So all you have to do is to count to twelve for each bread unit – et voila!

Really he said 12 grams of available carbohydrate, by which he didn't mean the total carbohydrate in any one food, but rather the amount the body could extract from the food for use.

So now you know!"

158

"Well go on, clever Dick, you do the maths: 12 into 72?"

"Easy peasy! That means an allowance of six bread units a day. Six bread units doesn't sound a lot, does it! It sounds even less than 72 grams!

I wonder how many grams we eat now?"

"We clearly have some unlearning to do," said Mum, smiling. "And, if we are really going to 'do a Wolfi', as you put it, we must allow ourselves to be guided by him.

The old boy, after all, has had nearly fifty years' experience with this way of eating. He is very sensitive to the wellbeing of his patients: he would be the first to draw a halt if he thought he had got it wrong about his medical advice."

"Fifty years without bread! Just think of it."

"You know very well that he didn't mean that literally," responded Mum a little curtly.

"The theory may be OK," I said, wavering a little in my resolve, "but to actually do it?"

I eyed the fruit bowl on the sideboard, which was piled high with oranges, bananas and kiwis.

"Here we are thinking of cutting carbohydrates, when fruit is supposed to be so good for us that we are told to eat it many times a day," I reflected.

"If you ask me – which I know you don't often choose to – I say there's a right muddle over it all," said Mum. "They tell us to eat mostly carbohydrates, and starches are fine but not if those starches are white and refined.

My gran ate white bread and lived until she was 93 in good health; mind you, she didn't eat much of anything."

"Did I tell you, Mum, how one day in class I asked our teacher whether sugar wasn't to be found in all those pieces of fruit we are told to eat daily?

She said yes and no! Fruit contained sugars, yes, but not sugar; that we were to avoid sugar, especially if it was white, not though other sugars, which we were to eat freely.

All round the classroom shoulders had shrugged, signalling that we neither understood nor intended to obey."

I could laugh as I thought of this now, but not so when I worked out one third of Uncle Wolfi's daily prescription and saw how small the portion of breakfast cereal was in my bowl.

"I could eat a day's worth of carbohydrate for breakfast alone!"

Disconsolate, I phoned Uncle and said as much.

"I'm quite sure you could eat a day's worth for breakfast, Sparrow. Have yourself a sensible breakfast and you won't need all that cereal!

Try scrambled eggs and butter with your toast, for instance and you'll soon see. I think you'll find that things will get easier as you get used to cutting down the carbohydrates."

"Scrambled egg on toast, did you say, Uncle Wolfi? You mean I can still eat bread?"

"If it suits, of course you can. In fact, at this stage you can eat whatever you like except . . . Didn't I give you only one proviso?"

Uncle was always getting me to use my brain.

"I can eat anything I like? So, theoretically, as long as it didn't contain too much carbohydrate in it, I could eat junk food all day long?

You see, I've worked out that I could have 4 bags of crisps a day and never eat fruit and vegetables again!"

"I trust without salt?" rejoined Uncle with dry humour.

"Oh Sparrow, words are such a problem: they get in the way of meaning! And you tease your Uncle by insisting on such an interpretation of my words!"

"I take the point", said I, justly reproved.

"The real point," continued Uncle: "is that if you cut down to six bread units a day, then it matters less what your meagre allowance consists of.

If you only eat 6 bread units a day, you cannot eat 10 units of pure sugar, for instance, which is what a lot of people do."

"And it's not just sugar", I said, remembering a previous conversation.

"Indeed no. Eating sugar, plus cereals, toast and jam, sweet drinks, potatoes and pudding can easily amount to 30, 40, or even 50 bread units, or BU for short.

In other words, since 6 BU a day will only be a small portion of your total food intake, you will not be eating the amount of carbohydrate that gets people into trouble with their health.

And Sparrow, never forget there is that rare commodity called common sense! Good luck with getting started!"

So saying, Uncle rang off.

Touché, Uncle Wolfi!

I told Mum what Uncle Wolfi had said.

"Now just you listen to me," responded Mum gravely. "I'm trying to tell you something!"

"I'm listening!" I said with my best air of attention.

"The other day your Uncle told me that very ill patients should be under a doctor's guidance.

For such patients, he himself reduced their carbohydrate intake very gradually and in stages, pausing at each stage until he was sure it was safe enough for them to proceed.

And there are some medical conditions your Uncle wouldn't think of dieting. Just remember that!"

"OK, OK," I conceded.

"So none of your talking of 'magic amounts' to your Great-Aunt Hilda, as though she could just 'do a Wolfi' all of a sudden and all would be well!"

Aunt Hilda was old, quite poorly and often bed-ridden. Mum paused to give time for this to sink in.

"In the 1970's, there was this American doctor who was getting quite trendy," she continued, "and who, in your uncle's opinion, was cutting down people's carbohydrate intake both much too far and much too rapidly.

So your uncle flew all the way to America to warn him of the dangers – I bet you didn't know that!"

"Did the American doctor listen to Uncle?" I wondered.

"I don't for a moment think so. It certainly did not change his advice to people, but that is not the point, is it?"

"You mean Uncle Wolfi had done his responsible bit?"

"Quite! Anyway, as I was saying, we must trust to your Uncle's experience and guidance until we have both been long enough on the diet to be able to judge for ourselves what works best for us.

Anyway, Wolfgang says that his low carbohydrate diet is, in practice, a very health-giving, health-maintaining and also a very comfortable way of eating. At least, that is the impression he hopes he has given us."

"We shall see, Mum, we shall see!"

19 COUNTING THE CARBS

I looked at Mum and Mum looked at me. It was time to take the plunge.

"All I know is that our eventual goal is to be six bread units a day each – that is if you are coming all the way with me?

Slowly, slowly, catch a monkey! What do you say, Mum?"

"Well, yes, especially as apparently we might be a bit tired at first, but not if we take it slowly enough. We are to shout if we come across or suspect any hitches."

"Uncle Wolfi says we can take as long as we like, so what do you say to three months or so for us to get started?" I asked, relishing any possible delay.

"It sounds a bit like procrastination to me!" said Mum. "Wolfgang also suggested that we needed to start by doing a little homework."

Not more homework, surely!

However, this preparatory work turned out to be fun.

First we needed to acquire kitchen scales that weighed in grams. Mum only had the old-fashioned sort with a big brass pan and massive weights for measuring pounds of damsons, plums and sugar in the autumn when we made jam.

Somewhere in the attic I'm sure I had seen an even older pair of scales – the sort apothecaries of old used for weighing out their potions by the gram. It had an upright pole and a balancing arm with a small brass pan hanging from either end.

I had liked the box of tiny weights you put in one pan to get it level with what you were weighing in the other.

Yes, that would do for now.

During the first couple of weeks, we were not to change anything and to eat exactly as we usually did.

By doing lots of weighing and measuring, we were to get to know the amount of carbohydrate we were accustomed to eat. Good to know where you start from, Uncle had said.

We soon set about with a will, doing all the weighing and measuring of all the items of food that we normally ate.

Mum and I worked out that our usual consumption of carbohydrate probably averaged about 30 bread units a day.

It was a far cry from six – and I personally didn't admit to the sweets!

I was glad that Uncle Wolfi had sent us two little charts to make this easier, because I could never make any sense of the 'nutritional information' on food packets and, in any case, fresh fruit didn't usually have labels.

"Come to think of it, doesn't one of his charts use bread units?" commented Mum.

"I must reread them", I said, feeling a little guilty that I had not been more thorough.

Mum now thought of a practical way forward. We would take two sheets of paper and put them up on the kitchen wall; on each we would draw a big wicker food hamper.

In the first, we would put the permitted food. From this hamper, we could freely help ourselves without the feeling that someone was looking over our shoulder!

Knowing how Uncle thought, we were not surprised that, apart from honey, he allowed us free choice of most kinds of food from the animal kingdom: fish, poultry or meat (the lean and the fat), eggs and animal fats such as lard and suet.

"Steak and kidney pudding with real suet – heavenly!" sighed Mum.

"Just a minute: the flour in the crust would have to go in the next basket, surely?" I queried.

"Bother!" said Mum.

We could have Uncle's notion of the best of dairy foods: cheese, fresh cream, butter and ghee ad lib (but not low-fat cheese or skimmed or semi-skimmed milk, not in this basket anyway).

Vegetable oils were permitted, though not preferred.

As to vegetables, Uncle Wolfi gave us a free hand with what he called watery salad vegetables. By this he meant those without much substance to them such as lettuce, tomatoes and cucumber, and also the leafy sort of vegetables.

We could partake freely of olives, mushrooms and courgettes. Uncle said their carbohydrates scarcely counted.

"Couldn't you just live happily on such a picnic basket!" exclaimed Mum dreamily.

In the second hamper, we would put all foods containing any appreciable amount of carbohydrate.

Uncle's table included, in descending order from the highest amount of carbohydrate to lowest: sugar, honey, cereals, dried fruit, bread, beans and lentils, potatoes, bananas, sweet corn and nuts, sweet fruit such as apples or pears, fresh or frozen peas and so on through various vegetables to yoghurt and milk.

The carbohydrate content of all those ready-prepared foods we ate, like pizza and pies had, of course, to be counted. But here the labels would help.

Sugary drinks must also go on the list. Uncle thought fruit juice best diluted and that even small glasses still counted, as did sweets and chocolate.

Come to think of it, this was the basket we did mostly live from. There was big change afoot!

Our next challenge was to work out what a bread unit actually looked like on the plate.

"Do you know what they did in Vienna, Mum?"

"No, how can I?"

"In those days, there was a popular type of bread roll called the Semmel. One of these rolls contained 24 g of carbohydrate, or two bread units.

For patients at the clinic, three bread rolls therefore constituted their whole day's allowance of carbohydrate!

If they ate anything else, it had to be of equivalent value in terms of carbohydrate.

Just think, Mum! We could have three bread rolls, plus anything we liked from the first hamper and, just like that, we would be doing a perfect 'Wolfi'!"

"Better still, we could have a half a roll at each meal, worth 1 BU a time, and top up each roll with another bread unit's worth from the second hamper! It was not a bad idea," commented Mum. "I'll go with the idea of equivalence."

We giggled when we first shared a medium-sized banana between us, as it seemed so stingy!

Half a medium-sized banana did, though, represent one bread unit for each of us, and from then on we retained that picture in our minds.

Likewise, one egg-sized potato was the equivalent of one bread unit, as was one tablespoon of cooked rice, two dates, one medium apple or one medium slice of bread.

In this way, we gradually assembled a mental picture gallery of one bread unit's worth of all the foods we normally ate.

As a reference point, Uncle Wolfi's table of equivalence definitely had to have a place on the kitchen wall to keep jogging our memories as to how much we could allow ourselves to take from the second hamper on any one day.

I needn't have worried about the content of the fridge. At first, it stayed the same.

Then, very gradually, I noticed a few changes but they were not disagreeable ones.

There was some new fruit juice 'with no added sugar' that I hadn't tried before. There were different cheeses and some pâté, and sometimes a lovely big egg and ham flan with very thin pastry. There might be two or three very tempting-looking steak pies, the sort she knew I loved.

I wondered where Mum was now doing the shopping! And there was more besides, with lots of variety.

Then it turned out that Uncle had said Mum should not just cut down on the sugars and starches but was to make sure there were attractive alternatives always available – and ones that would provide the right sort of nourishment both for her and for a growing lass.

So that was it!

Probably the biggest change in the kitchen department was that Mum started doing much more of her own cooking and got me involved whenever she could.

Packets, tins and many ready-made foods were less and less to be found in our house. Often, as I came down our drive on the way back from school, I would get a waft of a delicious stew.

That was definitely a plus!

Moreover, since the change was to be slow, at first we ate two potatoes instead of three or four, or we took only two slices of toast with our more traditional breakfast.

Previously we had chomped through the best part of a loaf between us, both of us being somewhat addicted to toast, especially with the addition of jam, honey or marmalade.

Experimentally, we allowed ourselves only a smidgeon of marmalade and found that, with a little extra butter, this was tasty enough.

One day, it might be only one slice of toast but there was no hurry for this.

The thought of marmalade took me back to my holidays by the lake all those years ago and of seeing Uncle Wolfi helping himself at breakfast time to a whole spoonful of marmalade with his cream and without any toast at all!

But then he was not a bread sort of man.

I must have pulled a face, for I remember him saying that, as to what to eat, he was only strict about what really mattered and that his patients were more satisfied and likely to persevere longer with his diet, if they had maximum choice as to what was on their plate.

"If people like marmalade – and I myself like marmalade – as far as I am concerned, they may have some marmalade!"

This memory now took on meaning.

I now learnt that Uncle Wolfi had warned Mum to see to it that I ate regularly, dividing my carbohydrate allowance fairly evenly over the three main meals.

If, at first, I needed to take the edge off my appetite between meals, I was to have appropriate snacks to hand. I will say that she was very good about this and I'm sure it helped.

Mum would provide me with cold sausage or a piece of cheese and, if she thought I couldn't otherwise avoid biscuits, she would supply me with a small packet of nuts and raisins or a small packet of crisps. Something about the lesser of evils!

Neither of us had yet tried the snack of putting unsalted butter on a piece of cheese, which Uncle had done when he first cut down on carbohydrate.

Somehow, just by taking a little less of things on the rationed list and by playing bread unit games, we managed to cut down to twenty units a day within a month.

Mum gave up sugar and milk in her coffee. Rediscovering the delight of pouring cream on the top of fresh black coffee and drinking the coffee through it, she said reminded her of the cafés of her youth.

I loved to see her taking such pleasure in something so simple.

So far, Mum felt fine and she was minded to continue.

In our attempt to 'do a Wolfi' – well, to start doing the diet – we had both taken slightly smaller helpings of rice and pasta as well as of potatoes, and had eaten more of the beans, meat, egg or cheese that accompanied such food.

For breakfast, if we didn't have bacon and egg, I ate beans on toast and Mum might have a cheese and tomato sandwich or natural yoghurt with just a few prunes.

Strange to say, neither of us felt the hungrier for eating less. To be honest, at this stage we scarcely noticed the reduction of bread units.

In another month, we had reached twelve bread units.

Mum had lost a few pounds and was looking good; she said she felt she could happily stay on that amount of carbohydrate forever. I think Mum only reduced further for my sake, as I still had the occasional wobble.

I was eating well and I noticed that I, too, was looking good and not so scrawny. For the most part, I had lost that feeling of incessant hunger, which had made me want to eat all the time.

So we persevered and were getting the hang of it. Instead of bananas, for instance, I got to love savoury 'fillers' like hummus on an oatcake or on crispbread.

Eating enough fat was not a problem for Mum, since no aspersions had been cast upon fat when she was young and it was only the last 17 years she had to undo. In fact, she was relieved by her return to a previous way of eating.

However, I needed a bit more coaxing, as I had never known other than a low fat diet. The pleasure of, say, streaky bacon was new to me; Mum grilled it until the fat turned brown and crisp and I soon took to enjoying it with beans or chopped and mixed with rice and tomatoes.

The fat on lamb and beef took longer for me to get used to, let alone appreciate, especially when the fat was hot.

Gradually, though, I discovered the delight of cold chops with salad. Eaten this way, I found that the fat on a lamb chop actually tasted really good, as did that on a portion of cold steak. It took a while, of course, but slowly, slowly . . .!

We had found that eating some fat with each meal – whether using olive oil in the salad dressing, tossing our veg in coconut oil or bacon fat instead of cooking them with water, or using any fat left from a roast in the gravy or in soup – somehow sustained us and stopped us hankering after carbohydrates.

We were still eating less overall and we didn't feel that we were eating any more fat than before, though that was difficult to know. As we were eating less packaged foods, we certainly ate less 'hidden' fat and less commercially changed fats.

One of our more bizarre discoveries, at least to my mind, was that of chips cooked in dripping. If we chopped two egg-sized potatoes into matchsticks and then fried them in beef fat, we got a surprising amount of French fries for 2 BUs – and so tasty! Amazing!

I learnt later that using dripping was the traditional way of cooking chips before the coming of commercial vegetable oils.

A friend with a bad gut said that the only way he could take chips without trouble was when they were fried in dripping. It appeared that there were still some chippies that fried that way in the North of England.

Wait until I tell Uncle Wolfi!

In general, I was quite well behaved as to 'doing a Wolfi' and I was beginning to feel more peaceful in myself and less excitable. However, my progress was not uneventful.

One Saturday, after a good breakfast and a tiny protein-rich snack mid-morning, I was feeling fine and quite complacent.

In a snack bar with friends, I ordered for lunch a baked potato with tuna mayonnaise. When it came to the table, it was the most whopping great potato I had ever seen: at a rough estimate it must have been at least eight bread units worth.

Naturally I ate the whole lot with my old gusto – I think it was my eyes that so tempted me, not my appetite – and I felt not a little full.

Within the hour, that old unbearable feeling of faintness mixed with desperate need for more food came upon me and I found myself suggesting ice-cream to my friends, who were eager enough.

By the time I got home, some two hours and two chocolate bars later, I was extremely crochety and immediately burst into a flood of tears.

Later that day, I phoned Uncle Wolfi. But when I had told him how I was no saint and confessed what had happened, he was not at all put out. I could almost feel goodwill being beamed down the phone.

"Sparrow," he said, "none of us can be a saint until after we are dead, so enjoy being a fallible human: forgive yourself and try again!"

It was wise advice. So I did forgive myself and did try again. No more impulse eating of spaghetti on toast, no more social eating of pasta with garlic bread and cake to follow, no more secret munching through a whole packet of peppermint creams all in one go!

Gradually it got easier not to overdo things, to choose a café where they did small platefuls or to take, say, just a small piece of cake at a friend's party or a small helping of fruit juice.

That way I could join in the fun but keep my system stable for I knew, though I didn't tell anyone, that Uncle was helping me to stop upsetting my controllers and so, if possible, to avoid real trouble in the future.

20   LAST VISIT

The following winter saw a second visit from Uncle Wolfi.   It was late October and he wasn't long back from Austria.

"What lovely warm hands you have, Sparrow" he said, as he took my hands and kissed me on both cheeks.

Warm feet, too, I thought, gratified that my progress showed. Mum, too, looked glad that Uncle had noticed.

"Thank you. We had a good journey back to England and just beat the winter snows," he said, as he later sat down to our evening meal.

Uncle Wolfi tucked heartily into the roast lamb, took plenty of the gravy and one small roast potato, politely declining the mint sauce and cabbage cooked with caraway seeds.

"Don't you like my vegetables?" I asked, a little hurt as I was getting to be proud of my newly acquired art of cooking them.

"Thank you, but personally I do not often eat vegetables. I tend to see plant food as an optional extra, but please feel free to enjoy them yourself."

I was pleased when he accepted the dainty dish of fruit salad that I had prepared for him and then helped himself to more cream.

"It worries my wife, so she puts a small glass of vegetable juice by my plate, which I dutifully drink!" he said, with the old twinkle in his eyes.

Uncle had aged since we last saw him. He was distinctly frailer and a little slower, his walks were shorter, bedtime a little earlier and, since receiving an infected tick bite walking in the woods near his home in Austria, one of his hips was now plaguing him.

But Uncle Wolfi was still upright and he still preserved his air of distinction. His lovable mixture of serious concern and realism was still apparent and his irrepressible humour and sense of irony seemed to keep him calm and unflustered as he got older.

We sat down round the bright fire and he looked us up and down approvingly.

"Na, und?" he asked, this time meaning 'how are you both and what have you been up to', whilst his approving glance meant 'I see the diet is having its effect.'

"I think we are quite converts!" said Mum.

"But I am not offering a religion!" said Uncle Wolfi, laughing. "And you, Sparrow, my special secretary? I was very happy with the last letter you helped me with: thank you."

I looked bashfully at the floor: pleased he was pleased.

"And many people liked the summary of my main book that we did together. I still can't work out how you are gaining such insight into my work but, at my club, my colleagues joke that at last they understand – what did they say – understand what I am 'going on' about?"

"What you are trying to tell them," I interpreted.

"But where are your hundreds of questions?"

"I am struggling with GIs," I confessed, glad of a change of subject.

Mum laughed: "When your gran was at school, GIs were what all the girls dreamed of, if only for the illicit cigarettes and the silk stockings."

174

"GIs?" asked Uncle, looking puzzled.

"Yes, all that about complex carbohydrates being OK for us to eat because they are slowly absorbed – it looks like your own teaching has been superseded," I explained.

"Ah," said Uncle nodding, but not without one of his special smiles. "Anything else?"

At this point, Mum disappeared on the pretext of doing the dishes.

"Actually, Uncle Wolfi," I said quietly, "Mum is going through what she calls 'the change' and since she's cut right down, she says all signs of it have completely disappeared."

"Good, good," he said. "I have many female patients who are very happy with the changes this way of eating brings."

I am not sure he had understood me about Mum, but it didn't matter.

"And about vegetables, some of my patients do not tolerate them very well – my GI patients, that is."

"Touché! Uncle," I said approvingly.

"Yes, my gut patients are not always thankful for certain vegetables nor, for that matter, are they always grateful for wholemeal bread and cereals."

"I read somewhere that fibre can hinder the absorption of nutrients," I commented.

"Not only that, but it can also speed the passage through the digestive tract. To some people this can, of course, be of help, but many of my patients find things go through them too quickly already and so need to avoid such rough things for some time, sometimes for life. And it does them good to do so.

I have letters from patients who had had very serious bowel troubles and who have been free for thirty or forty years by cutting down on carbohydrate and keeping wholemeal bread to a minimum, sometimes avoiding it altogether."

"It takes guts to stick to a diet that long," I said, awed at the prospect.

"It helps the guts, certainly," countered Uncle Wolfi with a knowing smile. "But, you know, it is best not to think of it as a diet, more a natural and permanent way of eating."

This mention of a natural way of eating gave me a nostalgic pang for my old way of eating and my hand automatically slid into my pocket in search of a sweetie, like it used to do.

That there were none there was a salutary reminder of my new way of approaching food!

"In general, though, Uncle, when can people put the carbos back in again?" I asked as casually as I could.

I had adopted this word so distasteful to Mum.

"If you mean when can people resume the excesses that caused them to be ill in the first place . . ."

"Well, I know that would be stupid," I interrupted somewhat sheepishly, as I had known full well what Uncle would reply. "What I mean is, once people are properly better, can they put up their carbohydrates a little?"

"Reports from my patients vary in this matter: some find they can eventually eat a little more carbohydrate and stay well, others have to remain on a low level in the long-term.

Once used to it, it is not arduous. Our bodies and our health tend to guide us and warn us with a nudge of our old troubles when we overdo things too much or too often."

Mum returned with a glass of wine for herself and for Uncle Wolfi. This he gratefully accepted.

"Cheers, Wolfgang, prosit!" said she clinking his glass.

"Prost!" said he, and we all three settled down for a long chat about the happenings of the intervening year.

"It is not as though we used to eat much junk food anyway and I always provided wholemeal bread," said Mum at one point, "but since we cut down to six bread units, which was over six months ago, I must say that that lass over there," she indicated me with a gesture of her head, "has been a lot easier to live with!"

"My point entirely!"

"Thanks, both of you!" I said, not very graciously.

"She is looking good, too," said Uncle winking at me.

"My skin is so different, Uncle Wolfi, if I cut myself I heal almost immediately and I'm sure I burn less easily in the sun."

"It figures," answered Uncle without showing any surprise.

"It is true," resumed Uncle, "that a wholefood diet with its so-called fibre-rich complex carbohydrates will fill you up more than refined foods do. Therefore, people may find they eat less carbohydrate anyway.

Health has been recorded as taking a downturn when refined foods, and especially such high carbohydrate foods as white flour and sugar, have been introduced to indigenous peoples. That they previously ate less carbohydrate – or, should I say, absorbed less carbohydrate – on their former wholefood diet is perhaps the main reason for this."

"Do you mean recorded by that dentist fellow who went round looking at teeth before and after such foods came into native diets?" I asked.

"For one," replied Uncle, "Stefansson for another."

"I read that dentist's book, you know!" I said proudly.

"Keep reading, Schatz! But always with your mind open or you might come to erroneous conclusions!"

177

"Well, cutting right down on carbos, whole or no, helped my wobbles," I confessed.

"In such cases," said Uncle, and I was grateful he made it impersonal, "it is essential to cut down carbohydrate from all sources to the level that stabilises the blood sugar mechanism – which I usually found to be about six or seven bread units, sometimes a little less."

"You mean cut down to a level that stops provoking all those overworked controllers and gives them a well-earned rest?" I said, teasing him a little.

He nodded, lapsing into thought.

"It must save on a lot of drugs," I muttered to myself.

"Naturally, the effect depends partly on the level of carbohydrate consumed," Uncle observed after a time, his eyes on the tapping thumbs of his clasped hands.

"You see, directly or indirectly, all the major controllers are involved in dealing with carbohydrate overload and are therefore all affected by it.

This, of course, can be detrimental to our health in so many ways – and don't forget we all have our differences!"

All the major controllers: I was glad I had got this bit right.

"Staying well partly depends on how well the controllers can keep defending people against the challenges thus posed and for how long, plus many other factors besides, such as strength of constitution, medical history, age, hereditary predisposition, level of physical activity and so on, as I think I mentioned.

This complexity of influence is, I think, why links with carbohydrate intake are so often missed."

I shook my head slowly in dismay: "I don't stand a chance then really," I said, thinking of the wider family.

"Of course you do! With such a family history as ours, you might have to be more careful than some and to avoid regular excesses, it is true. But how many times must I tell you that PREDISPOSITION DOES NOT EQUATE TO DESTINY: predisposition still gives you a chance and you, Sparrow, are already taking the right way forward.

My point was to give you an idea why such a surprisingly wide range of medical conditions are aggravated by an excess of carbohydrates and so may, in turn, respond favourably to sufficient carbohydrate restriction."

"Like your dicky hips, for example?"

"For example, like my dicky hips, as you call them. As I said, this includes medical conditions which don't obviously have any connection to what we eat!"

Uncle Wolfi looked up at me:

"And yes, it does save on drugs. A fragmentary approach can lead to the use of many different drugs whereas, by this simple dietary measure alone, a whole cluster of raised regulatory activity can be lowered and restored to normal."

"You mean the body is capable of its own micromanagement and we don't need to do it by giving all those drugs?"

"I mean that perhaps there would be less need for such measures if . . ."

"If we had more respect for the cuisine of our ancient relatives?" I suggested.

"Just so," agreed Uncle, smiling at the thought. "You see, drugs may adjust our operating system for a while, sometimes seemingly successfully but they don't get to the source of the problem: that is if the root cause is excess carbohydrate.

179

You see, Schatz, unlike with drugs, a restoration of health is genuinely promoted by actually reversing the carbohydrate effect through an appropriate way of eating," he concluded.

"Don't you give your patients drugs at all, then Uncle Wolfi?" I ventured to ask.

"As you know, I use both drugs and surgery as little as possible.

However, while patients with particularly severe medical conditions are adjusting to this new way of eating, they often need help over the transition time, even when carbohydrates are reduced very slowly as, of course, they need to be.

I have found that, under a doctor's supervision, a low level dosage of medication for a few months usually suffices to slow down or prevent any adverse reactions.

It is true that problems can come with very ill patients who read about this way of healing, get too enthusiastic and plunge straight in with a diet very low in carbohydrate. An ill body cannot always cope with such sudden change and the results can be very unfortunate.

In certain circumstances or in cases where I feel the diet to be insufficient on its own to bring about the requisite healing, I may have to recommend surgery."

Mum was listening intently and here she entered into the conversation.

"So slowly does it, restrict carbohydrates sufficiently and minimal use of drugs: this is all very interesting, Wolfgang. You see I have a doctor friend in Scotland who also uses drugs and surgery as little as possible, yet Walter's approach is very different.

Walter maintains that as long as you take little sugar and only eat wholefood, you'll probably succeed in avoiding all those diseases you talk about."

"In which case, Uncle, your own diet really would be superseded," I said, wanting to be provocative, "and all of us will be allowed more carbohydrate!"

"So, on the one hand, there's my old gran living healthily to 93 on white bread and cigarettes . . ." continued Mum.

"But, Mum, you did say she hardly ate anything and perhaps that's the reason? Not too much carbohydrate!" I broke in.

"You see I have an ambassador already," commented Uncle amused.

"On the other hand," persevered Mum, "there is my old friend Walter who advocates wholefood and, of course, there is your good self.

How do I square it all? After all, surely only whole is natural? And what about all those fats?" she pleaded

"Mum is thinking of trans, short, medium and long chains, saturated and unsaturated and even poly, high this and low that, let alone animal versus vegetable and fatty what's it."

"Thank you, Sparrow, I think I get the picture," said Uncle, before I could go any further.

"Perhaps, Wolfgang, you would like another glass of wine?"

"I thank you, yes."

Uncle Wolfi sipped his wine calmly and Mum put some more coal on the fire. There was a peaceful pause before anyone spoke.

21 HARMONY

"Now let us unravel all this," suggested Uncle at length. "If one avoids denatured foods, I feel one can dispense with all the side issues like calories, 'good' and 'bad' fats, even 'good' and 'bad' carbohydrates. Your throw, Sparrow!"

"I think Uncle would suggest that if, to be healthy, our Ice-Age relatives in Europe had needed to rely on, say, coconut oil rather than animal fat, then well . . . Well, they would have definitely died out and, as a consequeuce, there would be no descendents, i.e. no us."

"Uncle might add," said he smiling, "that, as to the various types of fat you just mentioned, Schatz, he feels the populace is being force-fed with quasi-scientific myths that they only half understand!

And the reason that Uncle seems to oversimplify things and talks just of 'fat' is to encourage you to look not merely at – what did you call them years ago – great splodges of paint? That is, to look not just at the current narrow fat fads, but to be able to see the bigger picture, the blue irises: in other words, at the important role that fat plays in our diet as a whole.

Back to you, Sparrow!"

"Well, as far as I can see, both you and Walter want people to stick to traditional fats that haven't been too messed about with, and to cut down on sugar to a minimum," said I.

"Correct!"

"And you also both say it is not just sugar. As far as health goes, Mum's friend says it is wholefood that counts, whereas you say it is the total amount of carbohydrate that counts."

182

"Good so far! Well done, but go on!" encouraged Uncle.

"Oh dear, I'll try," I said bravely. "Well, I know Walter is a fibre man and you are not always too keen.

Both of you reduce carbohydrates: you deliberately, Walter by default, as it were, because you can't eat as much rough stuff as refined stuff, and because the rough stuff goes through you pretty fast.

So that brings both you and Walter a bit closer, except that you don't like vegetables."

"Now be fair, Sparrow: I admit they have their place."

"But some of your patients are upset by them?"

"That's nearer the mark," murmured Uncle.

"And there was something I read about meat: that we shouldn't eat much of it because of farming methods?" I said.

"Then let us clean up the farming methods, not shun the foodstuff. What is it you say about babies and bathwater?"

"But do we have to eat meat in the first place?" interposed Mum, thinking of her veggie friends.

"No, one doesn't have to, and limiting carbohydrate will still be beneficial. However, I feel one should never underestimate the benefits of eating animal food, namely its suitability to our digestive systems and the essential nutrients it contains, which some people who don't eat meat may miss out on – not to mention the lessons of history," added Uncle, glancing at me.

"And the importance of beginnings? Oh yes, I shall enjoy sharing some of those lessons with Mum, Uncle Wolfi."

"There is a further snag that may come about when one limits the animal food to dairy foods," continued Uncle. "You see, dairy foods all come from female animals or female birds. If you then add nuts and seeds and grains, well these are also female-type foods, even if only from plants. By stimulating the female side too much, this can cause an imbalance between those controllers which influence the male and female side of things. Without meat to offer a balancing factor this, I feel, could lead to some serious problems both with our health and in society."

"Come to think of it, I read that our drinking water is like that, too," I said.

"Which would, of course, compound the problem." remarked Uncle, stretching his legs a little and thoughtfully shaking his head whilst gazing into the fire.

"Wolfgang, you were talking about Walter", said Mum gently, not wishing to disturb him too abruptly.

"Ah yes, Walter for whom I have a great respect – I did actually meet him and we did correspond."

"I didn't realise that, Wolfgang," commented Mum.

"Yes. In fact, he did me the honour of quoting me in his first book and I totally agree with him that food should be as natural and untampered with as possible. I have long felt so."

"But Walter is quite strict and you allow some naughties, Uncle," I objected.

"And you know the reason for that, Sparrow!" Uncle quietly reprimanded.

"I do, Uncle Wolfi. I'm sorry I interrupted."

"I also agree with Walter," said Uncle, getting a word in, "that keeping food whole may help avoid trouble in the first place though, in my opinion, this is by no means certain".

"Especially nowadays with the vogue for 'wholefood', that is ready-made or in snack form!" I added.

"Wholefood has become a veritable industry, Wolfgang, and those sugar-free dried fruit bars – so very sweet, I'm sure it is almost like eating pure sugar!" added Mum.

Uncle acknowledged Mum's comment and continued: "Yes, both Walter and I believe in the importance of diet in preventing various serious medical conditions in the first place.

However, when it comes to the actual treatment of those very diseases that traditional wholefood may well prevent, I feel that my diet adds an extra and essential dimension to the healing process and so, dare I say, tends to be more effective?

Certainly, my way is to cut down all carbohydrates – even whole ones – sufficiently for the body to initiate its own healing and then to keep carbohydrate low enough to prevent a return of the illness. I find 'rough stuff' inappropriate for certain conditions, as you know."

I sat silent but Mum was still ruminating:

"But, Wolfgang, rough stuff apart, couldn't you suggest the best of both worlds for your other patients, that is to insist on food, say, being unrefined, organic and whole, whilst still limiting us to 6 bread units?"

"That is absolutely fine – very good, if it suits."

"So why all this about 'eating what you like as long as'? Why all this choice?" challenged Mum.

"Ah, my problem is with the word 'insist'. Sparrow?"

"I remember you saying, Uncle, that you were strict only about what mattered most to people's healing and that was to limit the amount of carbohydrate they ate.

You said that if people had some choice about the rest of their food, they were more likely to stick to the diet.

And when I asked if I could eat junk food all day you said that fortunately junk food is usually so high in carbohydrate that I wouldn't be able to eat much of it anyway.

And do I remember you saying something about the occasional indulgence being good for you?" I asked hopefully.

At this, there came that familiar raised eyebrow.

"Oh Uncle Wolfi, it is so hard when all your friends are eating mountains of pasta!" I complained.

"Yes, Schatz, it is difficult to be strong enough to resist the indulgence of upping your carbohydrates, especially when people round you are eating your favourite starchy or sweet dishes, but that is not the sort of indulgence I meant, nor that I condone. Naturally, the odd lapse is forgivable – it is the person who lapses that will pay for it, as you know yourself.

Rather I was thinking that a small portion of something you love can make it easier to be strong against temptation."

"Like trifle?" I suggested. I knew Uncle loved trifle.

"Like trifle, for example. This is one reason why I seldom say that you must eat so and so, or you must never touch x, y, z – though your own body might say as much!

"You mean 'A spoonful of sugar helps the medicine go down?" I sang the question.

"You see, people are human," continued Uncle seriously and without heeding me, "and, as well as their tolerances and intolerances, they have their likes and dislikes.

Put it this way, what would you say Sparrow, if I said to you that your Controller No. 1 was still a bit out of order and so you must eat no ice cream at all for 12 months?"

"I would say: oh, sugar!"

"And you'd be quite right: it is indeed a question of sugar, blood sugar that is.

However, as long as the amount of, say, ice cream you eat is within your daily limit of six bread units – and preferably as yet only forms part of your limit, it is likely you will be able to eat some without unduly disturbing your blood sugar, whether or not it contains sugar per se.

Old-fashioned dairy ice cream has the advantage of having good traditional fat in it, too! So enjoy, bless you!"

Mum now went off to see about something. As for me, my yearning to learn more about Uncle's medical work quickly reasserted itself.

"Uncle, this evening you mentioned the word 'normal': restoring to normal a whole lot of disturbed regulatory activity, I think you said.

In your red book, you talk of all sorts of blood levels normalising and of all sorts of organs being a lot happier.

Do you think that the key to your success is that, in some way or other, the diet itself brings things in general back to normal?"

"Naturally, we are not sure these days what 'normal' is," said Uncle Wolfi both modestly and quite seriously. "It is some time since the Ice Age!

There are always exceptions, of course, and for different reasons, but my own findings with my patients are that my diet does tend to successfully bring things within the parameters that modern medicine recognises as normal."

"Sounds brilliant," I said in appreciation.

"Thank you, Sparrow!" Here Uncle chuckled to himself.

"And I don't think there is a medic who would dispute the desirability of bringing, say, our various blood levels within these parameters, though of course there are a great many who doubt that diet in itself could have such a wide-reaching effect – especially my own low carbohydrate diet!

Over the years, I think I have amply demonstrated otherwise, yet could I arouse much interest in it? No, I could not!

But then knowledge based on direct observation is, shall we say, somewhat undervalued in my profession.

Na ja! I remember spending many years traipsing from one university to another to try to get scientific studies instigated but, you know . . ."

"And still do?" I said, remembering well his detour via Cambridge on his last visit.

"Not so often nowadays, Spatz," replied Uncle Wolfi, with a touch of resignation to his increasing years.

"So people wouldn't listen to your secret, Uncle?"

"My 'secret', as you call it, is so far from the recommended guidelines that perhaps people didn't want to listen – it would, I think, upset too many apple-carts!"

"Well, both Mum and I feel the better for following your advice, Uncle," I said in genuine gratitude.

"Certainly we do," chimed in Mum, who came in just then.

"I'm very glad of it," said Uncle really pleased.

"So when things return – I won't say to normal – but at least to within these parameters, our controllers are co-operating again as they should and harmony prevails?" I added.

"That is so," said Uncle, nodding.

Uncle's hips were getting a little stiff from the prolonged sitting. It was time for a break and a potter. I put the kettle on.

Uncle Wolfi got up and Mum showed him our records for him to choose a little music.

Uncle chose a Mozart piano sonata played by a fellow countryman of his, to which we all three listened happily. And harmony prevailed that evening.

22 THE BIGGER PICTURE

"Uncle Wolfi, I was reading that book you wrote with your veterinary friend, the professor. We don't do biochemistry at school so most of it was over my head, but there was a point in that book that I wanted to ask you about," I said.

"Go on, please."

"Excessive stress is obviously detrimental to our health. Right? Well, you said that, in modern life, there were three main sources of excessive stress: namely a relative lack of exercise, mental and emotional stress, and carbohydrates.

Is that what you still think, Uncle Wolfi?"

"That book was years ago, Sparrow, and perhaps we should add pollution overload of various sorts. But yes, I still think carbohydrates a stress and a major one at that."

"I liked the bit about the three stages of stress: initial alarm, then a period of adaptation to that particular stress, then finally a breakdown from exhaustion and so an inability to cope any more with it.

Is that what happened with the Copper Eskimo when they first got the ship's biscuits? First, quickly pee out the extra sugar, then get used to it, then get our diseases?"

"In essence, yes: but it is also too simple and not the whole story. However, I agree that it is a very useful way of understanding, say, the recent surge in certain types of blood sugar problems."

"For instance, when Controller No. 1 gets so exhausted that medicine needs to be given?"

"A case in point," agreed Uncle, "but I would beware of imposing any rigid model on such a process. I myself think that the carbohydrate effect is wider than that model and often shows itself long before that final stage of exhaustion."

"Like when Controller No. 1 gets overactive?" I suggested.

"Exactly," said Uncle with approval. "Recognising early signs of carbohydrate overload in this and other areas would, if properly understood, point to sensible and effective ways of helping people change their diet before needing any drugs."

"One thing I read somewhere else, and which puzzles me," said I, "is that during the stage of adaptation, whilst they can still tolerate it, the stress factor – say carbohydrate – actually makes people feel better if they keep eating it.

Is that so, Uncle?"

"If the body's defensive line-up were in tip-top condition, yes, I imagine it could be so.

Sparrow, here you are preceding me into realms I have not yet entered.

One man can only do so much. You see, I was working as a loner who really needed a whole research team to carry his work further."

"Fair enough, Uncle, I'm sorry. It is not your line."

"As I said, one man cannot cover everything. I can see that you have been reading my 'Stone-Age' friend Richard's work. Good, good. Carry on, Sparrow!"

"There was one statement in your own book that quite blew my mind," I said, changing topic. "Your professor said that eating excess carbohydrate upset the internal regulation of all warm-blooded animals.

Can that be true, Uncle Wolfi?"

"Remember we do share a lot of our body processes with the other animals, you know," answered Uncle with amusement.

"But they give cows molasses and treat horses to sugar lumps!" I rejoined.

I was worrying whether this counted as excess and thinking back to what he had explained to me about my neighbour's blackbirds and their raisins years ago.

"And I read that they feed sugar to cows because they want to change the quality of the fats in the cow's milk in order to make it good for us," said I.

"It seems, having lost respect for the wisdom of nature's laws, we are losing our way," remarked Uncle sadly.

"But ALL WARM-BLOODED ANIMALS?" I persisted. "You mean that dogs, rabbits, robins, wrens and even giraffes can be harmed by eating too many carbohydrates?" I said stunned at the thought.

"It would seem so, but my professor, as you call him, has much wider research experience than I. Personally, I can only speak for humans – and perhaps hens," replied Uncle Wolfi in his ironic way.

"But based on my very long clinical experience, it is my conviction that excess carbohydrate definitely does adversely affect our own internal regulation.

In turn, this can lead to . . . but we've discussed all that so many times, just as we have the reasons for so many variations in people's response, let alone what counts as excess.

Suffice it to say that spotting signs of distress engendered by carbohydrate overload can lead to safer ways of treatment."

"Did I understand that both you and the professor agreed that if people reduced the stress of excess carbohydrate, then

192

the other two stresses would be less, well, less stressful?" I asked tentatively.

"I certainly found so. I noticed with my patients that, when excess carbohydrate was removed from their diet, a great many of their body systems did calm down.

This included the nervous system and my patients felt more peaceful in themselves.

Reduction of stress also showed itself in that people's bones and muscles, even internal muscles like the heart, tended to improve and strengthen, as did external muscles - and without special exercise. I had found that with my own body long ago!"

"And more resistance to infections?" I put in. "And wouldn't that help all of us when there are lots and lots of bugs around?"

"Indeed, it probably would, Spatz," agreed Uncle Wolfi, thoughtfully and humbly adding: "Less stress? Or should I say less stresses? Perhaps that is it?"

"Oh Uncle . . ." I burst out, but Uncle had more to say.

"My role has been to advocate the prevention of deleterious effects by the timely limitation of carbohydrate – and not just effects on our internal regulation, though perhaps they start there – and the mitigation of these effects by a suitable and health-restorative reduction of carbohydrate."

Mum had just slipped in quietly to join us, and was looking at us questioningly while Uncle Wolfi continued speaking.

"It goes without saying that fresh air, fresh water, shelter and companionship are all necessary for good health.

As for food," said Uncle turning to Mum, "what I'm trying to say is this: if trouble stems – however distantly – from an overload of sugars and starches, then only the actual removal of that overload will go to the root of the problem, giving a chance of lasting healing."

"So, to give our health a real chance, it all boils down to a simple message: STOP OVEREATING THE STUFF!" said I.

"As usual, I do not approve of your use of language, but the meaning is clear and the summary correct," retorted Uncle.

Mum was nodding in approval of Uncle's mild reproof.

Uncle paused and looked at us both.

"Best of all is not to overeat carbohydrate in the first place!" said he with his habitual chuckle.

"However, to get the message across in society generally, there first needs to be acceptance of the unsuitability to our physiology of a diet based mainly on carbohydrate, don't you think?" asked Uncle, looking at me.

"They need to see that what they are recommending is making us ill!" said I, looking at Mum.

"Secondly, there needs to be official recognition that carbohydrates can have adverse effects on the body, especially as regards the extensive ramifications to our health of the all too common overeating of them.

Once cognisance is taken of the carbohydrate effect . . ." Here Uncle broke off and rephrased what he was saying:

"Once they see the bigger picture . . ."

"Then at last something can be done about it!" I said finishing his sentence, clapping with enthusiasm. "And there will be a way – slowly, naturally – for peace, health and harmony to be restored to our bodies!"

I glanced at Uncle's face, which seemed to say 'if only!' He shook his head and merely said:

"For this to happen, Schatz, there is still such a long, long way to go!"

"At least, in this household, there are already two of us who are benefiting from your advice, not to mention the many thousands of your former patients.

Oh Uncle Wolfi, I really think you should be famous!" I said quite sincerely.

"Well, they haven't exactly given me a knighthood but, after what seems like a lifetime of swimming against the tide, I am beginning to get a modicum of recognition.

But, you know, it doesn't work like that. Just because you find something to be true – and you can show it in practice – does not necessarily dismantle a myth."

"You mean, for example, that finding something isn't so is not enough to correct a long-standing belief that it is so? But, Uncle Wolfi . . ." I added in naïve protest.

"Oh, I found that out long ago, Sparrow. Let me tell you a little story about the war-time," he said, settling himself more comfortably in his armchair.

"I was working on a way to save the lives of pilots in high-flying aircraft. Cabins were already pressurised but if for any reason this pressure failed at very high altitudes the pilots lost consciousness, which obviously was not propitious."

Uncle was shaking his head slowly and from the expression on his face I could tell this was dire.

"It was thought at the time that this loss of consciousness was caused by bubbles arising in the blood vessels from the change in pressure.

However, I was able to show that the bubbles only came later and that consciousness was lost immediately the pressure failed, giving the pilots no time to take remedial action.

My discovery enabled me to design a special suit that automatically inflated the instant pressure dropped. It was a short-acting device, such as is seen nowadays on astronauts working outside the space shuttle, only my own oxygen flask was worn on the leg.

But I think you both already know about my prototype of the space suit?"

Both of us sat silent, with our eyes fixed on Uncle.

"Yet here we are half a century later and I still read that it is bubbles that cause loss of consciousness.

The folklore of science is so difficult to shift!"

Uncle was gazing into the by now dying fire, slowly shaking his head as he thought of this.

"Perhaps it is the same with the work I did subsequently on carbohydrates?

So strong is the general belief that carbohydrates should predominate in our diet that my findings about the harmful effects of overload and the need for enough fat, though I have verified them, do not even dent modern nutritional folklore.

Plus ça change!" he said, shrugging his shoulders.

Then, spreading out his hands, Uncle added his familiar:

"Na ja, na ja! Yes, perhaps mere demonstration of a truth is seldom enough to correct belief, and any change in that belief trails years behind."

"Oh Uncle, and even I was trying hard for so many years not to believe you – in fact hoping to disprove your ideas. I'm sorry!" And I momentarily hung my head in shame.

"You were not alone, my dear." Uncle had never called me my dear, not in English anyway and it felt strange.

"But," I burst out, "thankfully I failed!" and flung myself into his forgiving arms.

"Yes indeed, seeing that something is true is seldom enough to alter belief," repeated Uncle Wolfi, patting my head just as in the old days.

"You mean people won't believe the truth, Uncle?" I asked looking shyly up at him.

"I mean that myths seem to gain a strength all of their own. Yet we mustn't give up on our work, must we, Schatz!"

Uncle Wolfi seemed accepting of this statement of how things operate. Yet I knew that Uncle had never given up hope of publishing a definitive paper that would open the eyes, if not of the world, then at least of the medical profession, that it might abandon what Uncle saw as its erroneous thinking and find its rightful path once more.

23   A PROMISE

It was the last time I saw Uncle Wolfi, but we by no means lost touch with one another.

When I was quite a bit younger, I had written a story simply called 'Uncle Wolfi' to tease him.

When he eventually got round to reading it – his desk was always piled high with papers and journals that must have been far more pressing for his attention – Uncle had phoned me to say how much he and Aunt Helen had enjoyed reading the story together.

His only comment was that I had made him out to be a far nicer person than he really was. So I tried again and I had now made him, at times, a little over-bearing, occasionally snapping at his 'little Sparrow'.

I also added in a lot of what I had since learnt.

After his last visit, Uncle had taken this new attempt away with him to read on the train. A few weeks later he rang me:

"Sparrow, I like what you have written a great deal and I especially admire your fanciful imagination."

"Poetic licence?" I answered in excuse, remembering his reply when I quizzed him about a literal 'life without bread' many years before.

"That is all very well, Sparrow, but from now on, I feel it would be best if I tell my own story," said Uncle decisively.

"I did my best," I protested. "Oh Uncle, I had to do it that way because they just don't know!"

"Who don't, Schatz?" said Uncle, softening a little.

"My friends, my fellow students. They don't seem to have a clue about how the body actually works or even where things are! I mean, I was at a yoga weekend recently: there were fifty of us and I was the only one who knew where my liver was! One in fifty, Uncle, I couldn't believe it!"

"I can believe it," said Uncle Wolfi, who by this time was smiling at the vehemence of my protestation. "You've written a good story and I enjoyed it. In its way, I suppose what you say is sound."

"I'm glad because my story is our story – it is about you and me, Uncle Wolfi, and the special times we spent together. I had such fun writing it all and, albeit a product of my 'fanciful imagination', I would like to do something with it.

The conversations I had with you taught me so much. They helped me get well and may help others to do likewise?" I suggested hopefully.

"I suppose such whimsical writing has its place and could, I think, be useful background for people unfamiliar with such matters. Do as you please with it, Sparrow."

It was as near as I was going to get to his blessing and I was thankful.

"So what would you like me to do, Uncle Wolfi?"

Uncle Wolfi considered for a moment, then said: "As I was saying, I feel I would like to tell my own story and to do it myself. Now, I would like to do this in English so, of course, I shall need your help. Perhaps, I could tell my story to you, and you could then write it down for me: what do you think?"

"What about 'Who's afraid of the big bad wolf?' It's a good title," I suggested, my imagination already running overtime. "You would be amazed at how many people feel threatened by the idea of 'cutting the carbs'. I know many of my classmates are afraid to even try."

"I will be amazed? You forget, Sparrow, that I have been helping people do just that for decades!"

"I repeat: I, myself, will do the telling and you will confine yourself to writing it down in good English. Agreed?

If you like, you can add to what I say from my books and articles or from what we have already discussed together, but you must show me every word you write – every word!"

"Oh, Uncle," I said, dithering a little. Then a thought struck me and I added eagerly:

"I know: I could interview you! I am old enough now to be working for a local newspaper. Yes, I'll pretend to be a reporter."

"No Sparrow, no more of your pretending games – this is for real."

"You have made yourself quite clear, Uncle," I said, noting his firmness of purpose.

"But you will write me my own story?" Uncle was again asking. "You can understand, can't you Sparrow, that I want to record in English my own memories of how I came to realise the detrimental effect of an overload of carbohydrate and how this changed the whole way I treated people for many of their illnesses.

You can understand, too, can't you that I want it to be <u>my</u> book and <u>my</u> story?"

"Yes, Uncle Wolfi, I can understand."

Recently, Uncle had been involved in a joint book in English on his medical work, in which Uncle felt that he had not had enough say. So I could quite understand that he did not want a whippersnapper like me with her own ideas getting in the way of his project.

"Will you do it? My story?" he pressed.

"Including your confessions?" I asked, somewhat cheekily.

"Yes, I know you will demand something of the sort from me," said Uncle laughing. "We will have to see about that! Na, und?" by which he meant: would I do it?

"Hand on heart, Uncle Wolfi," I replied, "as best I can, I will be your most true and faithful scribe, honest I will."

And so it came about that I had another exciting commission to fulfil. Uncle had said long ago that one day I might tell his story and so it was to be, though it was to take me many years and I was almost through university before it was finished.

Slowly, I put together fragments of a great many letters that Uncle had written in answer to a great many of mine.

I incorporated information gathered from old articles and books that Uncle had written, from our numerous phone conversations and from his endless reminiscences. Some of these he had related when he came up North to visit us.

Then there were the questionnaires, which I sent for him to fill in to make sure I had understood what he had said, and then asking the same questions again to crosscheck the answers just like a proper researcher. I was neither Uncle's Spatz nor his Schatz then, I fear!

During this time, I was full of the argumentativeness of youth and I came out with enough doubts and 'yes, buts' to try the patience of a saint let alone that of Uncle Wolfi.

However, Uncle did once admit that he actually appreciated my probing questions.

On the other hand, and perhaps not surprisingly, there were misunderstandings galore. This was sometimes because of difficulties with language and sometimes because of errors in his typing when, at his great age of over ninety, Uncle Wolfi abandoned his old typewriter and bravely tried to conquer the complexities of the modern computer.

Our tiffs and clashes were always made up in the end and, most of the time, we were very close and positive and made good progress.

The exciting story of Uncle's life and work did eventually emerge from my pen. It described the very essence of what anyone enquiring into his teaching and method most needed to hear – and yes, Uncle Wolfi did read and approve every word.

Alas, Uncle himself was getting ever older and I was too inexperienced to launch it myself at the time, as Uncle Wolfi hoped I would. Much to our mutual regret, that particular result of our long and challenging co-operation did not therefore see the light of day during Uncle's lifetime.

During the last few years of his life, Uncle Wolfi did receive recognition for his medical work. Honours just seemed to come pouring in, but he stayed as unassuming and modest as always.

"I myself don't need any honours", he said to me once, "but I'm glad of it for the sake of my work."

On one occasion, Uncle Wolfi was guest of honour in recognition of a new title that was being conferred on him. When refreshment time came, this pioneering advocate of a life with little or no bread – what was he handed?

Sandwiches!

Uncle must have appreciated the irony, though he said not a word. With a quiet dignity, Uncle Wolfi discreetly removed the outer layers of the sandwiches and ate the ham that was in the middle, carefully wiping his fingers on his napkin!

Uncle went on occasionally seeing patients until well into his nineties. During these last years, Uncle Wolfi and Aunt Helen continued to over-winter in London and to spend their summers in Austria.

I had my own life to lead, but Uncle and I still kept in regular touch by phone. Uncle Wolfi and I had our special way of communicating, born of long practice. He used to tease me, saying that I got 'under his skin' and that I knew what he was thinking, even if he had not yet said anything about it.

It was in this way that Uncle and I continued to be able to hold meaningful communications. Even when Uncle Wolfi was on his ebb tide, I would phone and tell Uncle what I was doing and I could tell by the precise timing of his laughter that he could understand me.

Towards the end, I contacted Uncle Wolfi and reassured him that I had every intention of bringing out our book, and I knew from the encouraging noises he made over the phone that he still wanted me to do so.

"And when they interview me, I'll tell them you have no magic wand, that your diet is no panacea but that oh, such a lot of suffering could be avoided by people sufficiently restricting their intake of carbohydrates.

I'll tell them that it is not just sugar that causes trouble, and that there is a way to help so many, many ailments.

I'll warn them not to ignore who we are, how we work or how we are made - or even who we were!

I'll pass on your advice about doing your diet safely.

I'll recount the many, many advantages of eating that way.

I'll tell them the good news that . . . that your wonderful diet is so simple, so easy, so nutritious and that . . . but I don't have to tell you, Uncle, do I – after all, it's your message!"

I heard a faint chuckle, followed by sounds of contentment when I then whispered down the phone:

"I will do it, Uncle Wolfi, I promise."

Old age was catching up with him and, having reached the grand age of ninety-seven, my remarkable Uncle Wolfi died during his summer stay in his native Austria.

'I depart as air, I shake my white locks at the runaway sun'

That poem again!

'But I shall be good health to you nevertheless.'

Yes, you will, Uncle, you will continue to bring good health both to me and to thousands of people.

Oh Uncle, I shall always remember you with gratitude and affection. And, dear Uncle Wolfi, perhaps is it time for your little Sparrow to:

'sound

your precious secret

over the roofs of the world?'

Postscript

My promise to bring out the book was kept.
As agreed, gone were the fanciful flights of
my imagination, the pond, the lake, the games
in his old garden and the lively conversations.
These were, after all, only a playful way of
presenting the many discussions in which
Dr Lutz and I explored ideas together.

I, Sparrow, was now Valerie Bracken and
Uncle Wolfi the real-life Dr Wolfgang Lutz
telling his own story through my pen in the
book My Life Without Bread: Dr Lutz at 90.

I had been a faithful scribe and in the book
can be found the information to which clues
have been given here, also an overview of his
life and work, references, notes and a list of
all the books and articles Dr Lutz ever wrote.

Meanwhile, I add here a short glossary of some
of the more playful terms used in this book.

V. B.

A SHORT GLOSSARY

Regulators / Controllers   The endocrine glands
Controller No. 1   Insulin
Controller No. 2   Growth hormone
Controller No. 3   Cortisol
Controller No. 4   Thyroid T3 & T4
Whole group of controllers   All the above + the sex hormones

Little cell engines   Mitochondria

Clinic for treating blood sugar problems   Clinic for diabetes

Gate-shutting   Insulin resistance

Help over the transition   Cortisone

Spatz (sparrow) Schatz (treasure)   Terms of endearment in German

The lot before us   Neanderthals

Experiment in New York   Bellevue Experiment

Impending doom   A state conducive to cancer

Friend Walter   Dr Walter Yellowlees

Friend Richard   Dr Richard MacKarness

G.I.s   American soldiers in the 1950s, glycaemic index and
gastrointestinal ailments

Medicated margarine   Cholesterol-reducing

That poem again   Walt Whitman's Song of Myself

That dentist fellow   Weston A Price

Your veterinary friend, the professor   Schole J

Three stages of stress   Selye H

A fellow countryman   Walter Klein

You are old, Uncle Wolfi   Adapted from Lewis Carroll

I would like to thank my family and friends, especially Sarah and Mark, for their help and encouragement whilst working on this book. I would also like to thank Charlotte Cornforth for her back cover painting of the mountain: Grossvenediger, Austria.

Made in the USA
Las Vegas, NV
19 March 2025

19818626R00115